Power and Conflict between Doctors and Nurses

Breaking through the inner circle in clinical care

Maureen A. Coombs

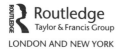

Routledge
Taylor & Francis Group

LONDON AND NEW YORK

First published 2004
by Routledge
11 New Fetter Lane, London EC4P 4EE

Simultaneously published in the USA and Canada
by Routledge
29 West 35th Street, New York, NY 10001

Routledge is an imprint of the Taylor & Francis Group

© 2004 Maureen A. Coombs

Typeset in Bembo by
Keystroke, Jacaranda Lodge, Wolverhampton
Printed and bound in Great Britain by
Biddles Ltd, King's Lynn

British Library Cataloguing in Publication Data
A catalogue record for this book is available from the British Library

Library of Congress Cataloging in Publication Data
A catalog record for this book has been requested

ISBN 0–415–30192–0 (hbk)
ISBN 0–415–30193–9 (pbk)

Power and Conflict between Doctors and Nurses

Health care is increasingly in the political and public spotlight, and organisational changes to improve patient care mean that the roles of doctors and nurses are under scrutiny. As a result, health care work is changing: the pre-eminence of the doctor is being challenged, nurses have increased decision-making power and interdisciplinary working is advocated. But how are these changes working in practice?

Power and Conflict between Doctors and Nurses is based on in-depth research in three UK intensive care centres and looks at the:

- development of contemporary nursing roles and recent moves towards greater interdisciplinary collaboration
- management of clinical practice teams
- power and influence of competing knowledge bases in clinical care and the ensuing conflicts in decision-making and practice

The book will be of great interest to academics and students of health and nursing, while the practice approach of the study makes it an invaluable resource for nurses and doctors looking to work collaboratively in clinical teams.

Maureen A. Coombs has held senior posts in coronary care, cardiothoracic and general intensive care. She is currently Consultant Nurse Critical Care at Southampton University Hospital Trust and holds a Senior Lecturer post with the School of Nursing and Midwifery at Southampton University. She has undertaken work in both policy and research with the Department of Health and professional associations towards the delivery of a contemporary critical care clinical service.

Intensive/critical care nursing/medical sociology/health

Contents

Illustrations

Figures

Tables

Acknowledgements

Ag filleadh ar do dúchais

The completion of this book, and of my Ph.D. research on which this is based would not have been possible without the support and help from many people, to whom I will always be extremely grateful.

Considerable thanks are therefore extended: to all staff in the sites who participated in this study, for their time and interest in this work; to my original supervisor, Dr Steven Ersser for his ability to guide and intellectually challenge; to Oxford Brookes University, Oxford and The King's Fund, London for their generous financial support for the original project; to colleagues who acted as critical readers and gave me encouragement; to my dear friends and family who have been there for me; and finally to those who watch over me.

The author and publisher gratefully acknowledge permission to reproduce material from the following publications: Coombs M., 2003 Power and Conflict in Intensive Care decision making, In: *Intensive and Critical Care Nursing*, June 19 (3) 125–35; Coombs M., 1998. Collaboration – working partnerships or sleeping with the enemy? *Nursing in Critical Care*; 3(4): 161–162; Coombs M., 2001. Towards collaborative and collegial caring: a comparative study. *Nursing in Critical Care*; 6(1): 23–27; Coombs M., 2001 Critical care: where care is critical *Nursing in Critical Care*; 6(3): 111–114.

Abbreviations and glossary

Adrenaline	Powerful drug given to stimulate/strengthen heart function
Acidosis	Acidity of blood and tissues indicating cellular dysfunction
Afterload	A haemodynamic measurement – *see below*
Amiodarone	Drug given to stabilise heart rhythm
Apnoeic	No breathing effort
Aspiration	Contamination of lung tissue with stomach contents
Asystolic	No heart beat
Bronchopleural fistula	Connection between lung lining and main air passage in lungs
Bronch.	Bronchoscopy – tube passed into lungs to view lungs
CABGx2	Coronary artery graft – cardiac surgery
Cardiac arrest	Patient collapse with no pulse or breathing
Cardiothoracic	Heart and lung speciality area
Cerebral infarcts	Bleeding/clot in brain that may result in brain damage
Chest drain	Tube inserted to re-expand lung
Cochrane	Evidence base medicine database
Consultant	Consultant grade medical staff; consultant nurse/other consultant practitioner grades not introduced into the NHS until after study was completed
CPR	Cardio-pulmonary resuscitation
CT scan	Computerised tomography scan – head scan
D and E grade	Staff nurse grade
Dry them out	Drugs administered to increase urine output
EBS	Emergency Bed Service – a national intensive care bed bureau
ECG	Electrocardiogram – heart tracing
Endoscoped	Procedure where flexible camera placed into body
ETT	Endotracheal tube – breathing tube
Extubation	Removal of breathing tube
Femoral pulse	Major pulse felt at top of legs

Fill	Administer intravenous fluids
G grades	Sister/charge nurse grade
Haemodynamics	Range of measurements taken to indicate cardiac function
Haemofiltration	Form of dialysis to support failing/failed kidneys (filtre)
HDU	High dependency unit
Hypotension	Low blood pressure
ICU	Intensive care unit
ICS	Intensive Care Society (medical association)
Inotropes	Drugs to support the blood pressure and cardiac function
Intravenous fluids	Fluids administered into a vein, as opposed to taken orally
K	Potassium
Labs.	Laboratory tests – biochemistry, haematology, immunology
Macindoes	Theatre instruments
Mentee	Student being supervised by a mentor
Midazolam	Sedative drug administered intravenously
Morphine	Analgesic (pain killing) drug
NAD	Nothing abnormal detected
NDU	Nursing development unit
Needs of elimination	Term used in nursing framework – concerned with bowel care
Obs.	Patient observations recorded on a chart
Output (cardiac)	Cardiac function or major pulse felt for in an arrest
PCV	Pressure controlled ventilation – mode of ventilation
PEEP	Respiratory support measure
Pre-oxygenating	Practice of administering 100% oxygen prior to procedures
Pressure support	Respiratory support given through ventilator
Propofol	Anaesthetic drug administered intravenously
Pulmonary oedema	Fluid in the lungs
Pumps	Patients having undergone cardiac surgery
RCN	Royal College of Nursing (nursing professional body)
Rescussed	Resuscitated
Sedation score −2	Patient responsive to deep painful stimuli – local policy
Septic	Septicaemia – infection in the blood
Senior Registrar	Medical grade directly below Consultant
SHO	Senior house officer (grade of doctor)
Support	Inotropic support – drugs to support functioning of heart

Swan (Swan Ganz)	Pulmonary artery catheter – invasive cardiac monitoring
Tracheostomy	Incision made in neck to ease the work of breathing (trachy)
User directorates	Clinical units sending patients to intensive care
Ventilator	Breathing machine
Volume loading	Administering intravenous fluids (volume)

Introduction

The writing of this book has been driven by the challenges facing clinical teams working within an ever-changing health service in the United Kingdom (UK). Increased consumer interest in health and illness, together with sustained political concern about health care, has had a massive impact on the health care services. The resultant workforce and organisational changes have brought developments in health care practice and role into sharper focus.

Health care is being increasingly placed under a spotlight, and the roles of nurses and doctors, among others, are being scrutinised. Traditional health care roles and scripts have been well rehearsed and firmly established, leading to customary practices and working patterns. Historically doctors have held centre stage, but this is now being challenged by acknowledgement of the contribution that others can make to health and social care.

Current health policy has provided frameworks for development of the National Health Service (Department of Health (DoH) 2003). Fundamental to this progressive vision is ensuring that patients act as the focal point for health care processes, and that patient care needs are serviced by effective clinical teams at every level of the health care organisation. At the heart of this modernisation programme is making maximum use of the skills and talents of the entire workforce. This is seen as central to an efficient, patient-centred service, and requires professional barriers between health practitioners to be broken down. If this is to be achieved, roles, relationships, behaviour and structures within the health service will need to be transformed: this issue is key to this text. Using the analogy of drama, an approach that is more extensively adopted later in this book, it is timely to explore further the roles of nurses and doctors, and find out where on the clinical stage, front or back, they really play their part.

The book is concerned with how doctors and nurses work together to make decisions within the clinical practice setting. It has, as its particular focus, the way that knowledge and roles are used within the decision-making process in the delivery of health care. The dominant power base is exposed, and the conflicts that this produces for both medicine and nursing are explored.

Whilst the attention of this book is on medical and nursing staff, it is important to note that these comprise but two groups of the health care personnel required to deliver health services. In describing the specific contributions of medicine and nursing, I am not ignoring the involvement of other health care staff, but simply stating my principal interest in this area and thereby rendering the depth and breadth of this text manageable.

I have been a critical care nurse since the early 1980s. During that time I have seen a great change in the treatments offered to the critically ill, and in the equipment available to support and monitor patients. This has required greater knowledge and skills to be acquired by all critical care practitioners, and these have resulted in changes to clinical roles, and to the way in which clinical teams function. Throughout my professional career I have experienced and witnessed reactions to such developments. Whilst I have had strong, positive experiences of close working and mutually respectful clinical teams, I have also been part of fragmented groups where, at times, it has seemed more like a battlefield than a clinical field. I have been left with an overwhelming impression that new ways of working adopted across health care teams have not always been accompanied by new working relationships.

The importance of successful team working at all levels of patient care delivery continues to be emphasised in health policy (DoH 2000a, 2000b, 2001b), and remains central to my personal philosophy. I believe that neither tribalistic nor egotistic behaviour will produce harmonious team working, with its concomitant positive impact on effective patient care (Knaus et al. 1986). For me, it is crucial to understand how doctors and nurses perceive team working, and the roles within the clinical team. From a basis of this understanding, factors that affect access to, participation in, and influence on health care services can be explored.

No one discipline operates alone in a health care vacuum. The nature of contemporary health care mandates a team approach. Yet, despite the fact that nurses deliver 80 per cent of all direct care (Royal College of Nursing 1992), nursing has traditionally been invisible in health care decision making and ignored by health care policy makers (Masterson 1994). Nurses continue to operate in a 'black hole' (Robinson 1997, p. 251). With the shifts in clinical roles and professional boundaries that have occurred over recent years, it is timely to study what impact, if any, this had had on how clinical decisions are made.

Whilst this book centres on how health care teams work together in order to make decisions in clinical care, it is impossible to analyse this across all health care settings. To enable an exploration of this in depth, I have used the clinical environment of intensive care. I contend, later in this book, that this is one clinical environment where, by the very nature of the clinical speciality, doctors and nurses are required to work closely together.

Two key domains provide focus for this book. The first is the interaction between medical and nursing staff at the interface with the patient. Here, patient management decisions form the focus of study. The second area is the interaction between nurses and doctors who, together with managers, run the clinical service. Through observation of activity in these two areas, the ability of both nursing and medicine to influence and contribute to clinical decision making is explored and examined.

As I have stated, health care policy, developments in technology and workforce issues have all been key in changing roles within clinical teams. These themes provide the focus for the first two chapters. I will demonstrate that nursing has become the major adaptor to such change: therefore, the recent evolution of the nursing role is the topic of Chapter 1. The first main function of the chapter is to present a contemporary overview of nursing role developments. The fundamental significance of economic drivers and health care workforce shortfall is highlighted, and the consequences for the nursing role are discussed. The second aim of this chapter is to illustrate such role developments through an exploration of the clinical context that underpins this book. The development of intensive care – and the resultant development of the nursing role – is therefore presented.

Chapter 2 acknowledges the role of the wider clinical team in decision making and details the nature of working relationships in health care. Through use of the nursing and sociological literature, with specific exploration of interdisciplinary working and collaborative practice, an understanding of how doctors and nurses work together is achieved. Chapter 3 explores the final subject that sets the scene for this book. This is concerned with how local clinical service provision is managed. The interface between managers and health care practitioners is reviewed through examination of general management in the National Health Service (NHS), and the relative standing of managers, doctors and nurses within the service delivery process is presented. The specific profile that nurses hold at this level of decision making is explored through discussion of the nursing contribution to the health policy process.

The following two chapters then introduce and describe the study and study settings on which the book is based. In Chapter 4, a brief overview of the ethnographic approach adopted and the data collection methods are given. To help the reader judge the validity of this work, details regarding data management and analysis are laid out, together with the actions taken to preserve rigour in the work. One of the challenges of undertaking the original study, and indeed of writing this book, is that I do not consider myself to be a social scientist nor a health care researcher in a purist sense. I am a practitioner. I have written this book to add to the social science health care literature, but I also want this text to be read by, and be accessible to, other health care practitioners. For this reason, Chapter 4 is longer than one may anticipate in such a text, and has a deliberate pragmatic element. This chapter explores some of the challenges I experienced when researching in my clinical field. It includes descriptions of gaining access to the study sites, and managing the fieldworker role. Using lived experiences that occurred during the fieldwork, the chapter concludes with a reflexive consideration of the complexities of the research experience. Chapter 5 provides greater detail about the study sites, and outlines the key areas in which decision-making data in the field were collected.

Chapter 6 explores a key issue that affected how doctors and nurses worked together to make clinical decisions. Using clinical examples, the ownership of different domains of knowledge by nursing and medicine is explored. It will become evident that there are shared and discrete areas of knowledge that are used by both medical and nursing staff. There is also discussion on the hierarchies of knowledge that exist and the impact of these on how decisions are made in intensive care. In Chapter 7, I discuss the divergent roles adopted by medicine and nursing in the decision-making process. Through this, the traditional role boundaries and definitions are, to some extent, challenged. Whilst it is clear that historical role perceptions are being questioned, it will also become evident that the influence resting with specific areas of knowledge or professional groups is not substantially changing.

Chapter 8 investigates this further through an exploration of power and conflict in the relationship between doctors and nurses. To reveal the complexities of this situation, I draw on Goffman's (1959) work and use a dramaturgical perspective to map elements of knowledge, roles and power involved in decision making in intensive care. Through mapping the public front stage and hidden back stage work, together with the official and unofficial roles of clinical decision making, the contributions of both medicine and nursing to decision making is established.

In Chapter 9, I draw the key themes from this book together and compare them with the aspirations, set in current government policy, for greater team working to ensure quality health services are delivered. I suggest that some salient lessons are to be learnt if the rhetoric of today is to be converted into the reality of tomorrow.

Writing this book has been the culmination of six years' work. Much thought has gone into its structure and content. I have written the book so that it can read as a continuous piece of work, or as stand-alone chapters. Similar to Allen's work (2001), it is a text that can be read at several levels. It can be given a substantive reading in order to understand everyday work processes in clinical practice; it can be read for its theoretical and analytical content in applying sociological theories to provide new ways of conceptualising medical and nursing roles in clinical decision making; and it can illuminate the use of ethnography in researching health care practices.

When I started the study on which this book is based, team working was an important political issue. This situation has not changed. The book is published in an era of continued turmoil in health care provision. All practitioners involved in care delivery have been challenged to change their practice, and develop their roles in order to make the best use of all available resources (DoH 2000b). This book has grown from consideration of the contemporary nursing role, and concern for an equitable team approach in the delivery of health care. The purpose of the text is to promote a critical awareness of the contribution of all team members to clinical decision making, with the call for alternative strategies to facilitate more effective team working in the clinical setting.

Chapter 1

Nursing role developments

Contemporary perspectives

This chapter explores key issues that have impacted on the nursing role in the clinical setting. Since the early 1960s, there has been great change in the content of medical and nursing work. Such change has occurred as a result of technological, professional, political and more recently, economic pressures. The fact that health care service workload continues to increase, is undeniable. From 1990 to 1998, acute activity in the UK rose by 38 per cent, and emergency admissions rose by 28 per cent from 1992 to 1998 (Buchan and Edwards 2000). This has resulted in an ambitious employment strategy (DoH 2000b) at a time when recruitment and retention of medical and non-medical health care staff is problematic (Caines 2001). This situation is not unique to the UK, with similar trends being noted worldwide (World Health Organisation 2001). Whilst all health care staff have been required to re-consider the remit and content of their work activities, it has been nursing and other non-medical staff who have predominantly developed their roles in order to meet the increasing service demand.

In this chapter, the impact of such pressures, at a time when the nursing profession is pushing its academic, clinical and professional boundaries, are explored, and the responses made by nursing to such changes are discussed. To illustrate the key issues raised in greater contextual depth, I will introduce the clinical field of intensive care. From examination of developments within this specialism, I make explicit the influence on the nursing role. Through this section, I hope that the reader will also become oriented to the specific clinical environment that acts as the central focus of this book.

Developments in nursing: a reactive or considered response?

In this section, a contemporary review of clinical role developments is undertaken encompassing both national and international perspectives. This review will demonstrate that there is clear evidence about the drivers for workforce developments in health care and that there remains much confusion about the developing role of the nurse *per se*. Several issues will be clearly evident: that nursing role development is currently occurring at an unprecedented rate and that, therefore, the boundaries of nursing are highly dynamic.

Historically, nurses have been striving for professional status since the end of the nineteenth century and this has been a focus of nursing debate (United Kingdom Central Council (UKCC) 1986). Discussions about the fundamental nature of nursing, and the nature of the nursing role were key areas in these discussions. Traditionally nursing role developments were described as expanding or extending practice (Pearson 1983; Reid 1998). Role expansion was linked to the development of nursing as a discrete service and built on the tradition of nursing managed through nursing autonomy and self-determinism. Role extension was used to describe roles developing beyond the traditional nursing boundaries, and oriented towards the work of other professional groups.

Demand for improved health care services, the increasing clinical component of nursing work, and the large numbers of nurses undertaking work previously considered within the remit of doctors (Casteldine 1991) were key issues precipitating role development. In the 1990s there was a proliferation of specific nursing role developments impacting across the health service. In the UK, the clinical nurse specialist (CNS) role was one of the earliest nursing role developments (Casteldine *op. cit.*). This role was initially established within the specialist clinical areas of infection control and intravenous therapy at the Royal Marsden Hospital, London. Many hospitals emulated the same medical speciality model, and nurses began to undertake work that doctors had previously performed. Clinical nurse specialists were identified as either being those who were technically oriented (role extension), or those who had developed a broader, more in-depth nursing knowledge base (role expansion).

Publication of the UKCC's *Scope of Professional Practice* document (UKCC 1992b) was seen by many to be the zenith of this era (Paniagua 1995). Through re-enforcing individual practitioner responsibility and professional accountability, this document was seen to liberate nursing practice (Redfern 1997) and effectively make redundant the terms role expansion and extension. However, this was published at a time when reduction in junior doctors' hours was being discussed. As a result, there was concern that the impetus for nursing role developments continued to be directed by, and dependent on, medicine (Dimond 1995).

The reduction of junior doctors' working hours was achieved through the transfer of tasks traditionally undertaken by the junior doctors, to others, most notably nurses (Walby and Greenwall 1994). This resulted in a profusion of new nursing roles including the development of the nurse practitioner role, for example in neonatal intensive care (Dillon and George 1997). It is clear that many such substitution and innovative roles now exist (Masterson 2002).

Despite this abundance of nursing roles, there was continued confusion about role definition, and an absence of understanding on the nature and purpose of these roles (Casteldine 1996). This is perhaps most clearly illustrated using the exemplar of advanced nursing practice in the UK. As originally perceived by the

UKCC (1994), advanced practice was distinct from specialist practice, and embodied in an expert nurse with developed political, professional and leadership skills.

The confusion concerning advanced and specialist practice was clearly demonstrated in a survey by McGee *et al.* (1996) on specialist and advanced nursing practice. This study utilised a self-administered questionnaire circulated to all senior nurses at trust board level in 371 trusts within England. The findings demonstrated that nursing role developments were diverse, multi-faceted, and perplexing. There were concerns about lack of understanding on specialist and advanced practice; lack of national agreement on the use of titles; and confusion on role responsibilities and remuneration of these posts. In response to such debate, the UKCC issued a position statement on advanced practice (UKCC 1997). Whilst offering these general guidelines and principles, the UKCC did not produce any further prescriptive policy.

There has been similar confusion and problems about nursing role developments within other countries. In North America, the initial development of the clinical nurse specialist role evolved in the 1930s from a nursing model of care (Hamric and Spross 1989). The nurse practitioner role, first recognised in 1963, developed in response to problems in the delivery of medical care (DeAngelis 1994). Role definition in North America has greater clarity, but practical difficulties exist in enacting role function due to the nature and working of the health care administration system. State terms of licensure, certification, remuneration and specific practice rights (drug prescribing and patient admission rights) vary across states causing practical and organisational role problems (Spatz 1996).

Medical staff shortages have also been strong drivers for specialist nursing roles in Australia. Sutton and Smith (1995) were critical of economic influences on nursing role developments. Through a review of the literature, together with anecdotal discussion with nurses, Sutton and Smith (*op. cit.*) argued that advanced practitioners should be developed to meet the personal needs of the client through the use of advanced holistic nursing skills, rather than meet medical agendas. By adopting this approach, it was suggested that nursing could determine a model for advanced health care practice. It is clear that the influence of medicine on nursing role developments, and the ability of nurses to direct these developing roles, are issues that nurses are experiencing at an international level.

The specialist nurse practitioner, the advanced nurse practitioner and more recently, the Consultant Nurse have all emerged as discrete nursing roles within health care. These roles are in different stages of formalisation and are all concerned with the adjustment of boundaries for the development of future practice. All require a more developed knowledge base, a higher level of judgement and decision making in clinical care, together with a responsibility to develop and shape policy and practice (Wallace and Gough 1995).

Much has changed since the inception of the NHS in 1948. As technology has developed and medical knowledge becomes more advanced, more treatments are available to sicker and older patients. As a result, greater staffing and financial demands have been placed on the health service. Successive inquiries have been undertaken by the UK government to ensure the productivity and cost-effectiveness of the service. The most revolutionary of these was the NHS and Community Care Act (DoH 1990). This introduced the internal market into health care. Whilst the impact of this review on the organisational health care structure is discussed in Chapter 3, its impact on the delivery of the service is my focus here. Through the drive for cost efficiency, new concepts were introduced into the NHS including skill mix review, role development and re-engineering of the workforce.

Such new initiatives have become all the more centre stage with the increasing concern about the insufficient numbers of doctors (Royal College of Physicians (RCP) 2001) and the need to implement new working patterns to meet the European Union Working Time Directive. Mather (2001) believes that meeting this legislation that aims to improve the health and safety, and working lives of employees, will have a profound impact on the structure of hospital life. This will either occur through positive impact with improved patient care being delivered by less tired doctors, or through a negative impact with a reduced continuity of care as a result of the reduction in the hours that a doctor is available. The RCP (2002) asserts that the increase in workload, decrease in trainee hours, and the resultant difficulty in obtaining locum cover has led to a demoralised workforce that is under continued pressure to cope with increasing work demands. This morale problem has impacted on retention both within the medical profession, and at medical trainee level (Goldacre 1998). Concern about sustaining the medical workforce has been further highlighted in the consultation paper on medical training (DoH 2002).

Some nursing role developments are clearly prompted by insufficient numbers of doctors. Even with an adequate nursing workforce, it is too simplistic a solution to assume that the majority of nurses want to take on medical activities (Medical Workforce Standing Advisory Committee 1997). Even if nurses wanted to develop in this way, there would still be a need to recruit and retain nurses in the NHS to undertake nursing duties. As outlined in the *NHS Plan* (DoH 2000b), the UK government is looking for 7,500 more medical consultants, 1,000 more specialist registrars, 6,500 allied health professionals and a total of 20,000 more qualified nurses. It is therefore important to recognise that workforce supply across health care is a key problem.

The role development debate is driven by the need to deliver a non-fragmented service, and to clarify the position of nursing within this. As this chapter has demonstrated, there is a resultant tension between regulating bodies, employers, practitioners and professional organisations (Frost 1996). However, the most profound challenge rests with the nursing profession and its ability to determine role boundaries to benefit and safeguard the patient, but without a fundamental shift in the nature of nursing.

Nursing has to respond and adapt to health care changes, and to develop nursing practice to meet a needs-led service (DoH 1993). Nursing may wish that this be as a direct response to clinical or patient population requirements, but in reality such developments have been sanctioned due to a growing realisation of organisational and workforce constraints.

Nursing role developments may be underpinned by an ethos of innovation and a drive for patient centred services, but health services can only be delivered by the numbers of staff available. In the current climate, where the predicted workforce growth required until the 2020s is estimated at 300,000 (HM Treasury 2002), and where radical change in health care staffing will be required in order to meet European Working Time Directives (DoH 2002), role substitution by nurses is a reality.

The intensive care environment

Change in health care roles has been witnessed across the health care spectrum and this has influenced how medical and nursing practices are enacted in all clinical areas. The exploration of clinical decision making throughout every health care setting was beyond the scope of this book. The specific clinical area of intensive care was chosen as the focus for this book. I made this decision, first, because of the evolving patient management treatments in intensive care and the fundamental nature of intensive care work. In order to explore how doctors and nurses work with each other, a clinical area had to be chosen that presented opportunity for such doctor–nurse interactions to occur. In intensive care, there is a nursing presence at the patient's bedside and medical support on most units, throughout a twenty-four hour period. The nature of the patient's illness in this environment necessitates a specialised nursing role to manage patient therapies, and a team approach to co-ordinate treatments.

Second, at the time of the study (1997–2000), there was increasing UK government scrutiny about the delivery of intensive care services. This resulted in the publication of several key policy documents. The first document (DoH 2000a) was the findings of an interdisciplinary expert group to radically modernise the delivery of critical care services. A subsequently published document *The Nursing Contribution to Provision of Comprehensive Critical Care Services for Adults* (DoH 2001a) presented the specific work of the nursing sub-group that fed into the 2000 publication. The publication of this nursing document was, in itself, a demonstration of the position and standing of nursing in this area. A key theme in both these policy documents was the need for partnerships between professions and specialities. Several key initiatives were introduced into the NHS as a result of these publications. Using the principles of equity of patient access, parity in standards of care, flexibility in clinical roles, and the concept of critical care networks and outreach teams were introduced. Such developments gave opportunity to develop new roles and teams in intensive care, with a concomitant opportunity for further nursing involvement in clinical decision making.

The final reason for undertaking this work in intensive care was that it was my home environment. As stated in the introductory chapter, the original purpose of this work was to understand my own clinical milieu better in order to work within, and across, all health care disciplines more effectively.

The specialist clinical units of intensive care are a relatively recent medical phenomenon. To understand the nursing role within these areas, and the nature of the environment within which this research is located, I present a historical perspective of intensive care. Through this, I will demonstrate the impact of technological development on intensive care units. From this, the impact on medical and nursing work can then be understood.

The importance of a designated area for close observation of acutely ill patients was initially recognised in the nineteenth century. As identified by Nightingale: 'It is valuable to have one place where post-operative care and other patients needing close attention can be watched' (1863, p. 25). Initially evolving from units located near to theatre, the concept of intensive care units was further developed during the Second World War. During this time, temporary military intensive care surgical units, trauma hospitals and 'shock wards' evolved (Noc and Weil 1996). In these designated areas, patients with multiple injuries and major surgery were treated. Permanent designated areas for critical care were finally developed in the 1950s.

Intensive care medicine has evolved as advances in technology and the ability of medicine to treat and support disease, have occurred. For example, the development of automated bedside monitoring (electrocardiograms and invasive pressure monitoring for cardiorespiratory functioning) has radically changed the capabilities of intensive care. Blood banking techniques (Fantus 1937) and the development of haemodialysis towards the end of the Second World War (Kolff 1947) both significantly reduced patient mortality. The onset of the poliomyelitis epidemics in 1951–1953 radically changed the technology and uptake of intensive care. The introduction of positive pressure ventilation through a tracheostomy reduced the requirements for medical students to be employed in manually ventilating patients. Medical developments of electrical defibrillation and cardiac pacemakers (Day 1963), and the advent of effective antibiotic therapy further shaped intensive care practice (Weil et al. 1964).

The location of such diverse technical therapies in one specific area led to the intensive care unit becoming the 'hospital's hospital' (Oh 1996, p. 12). The proliferation of generalist intensive care units have since evolved into specialist units including neonatal care, cardiac and cardiothoracic, renal, neurological, and paediatric intensive care units. All of these units are encompassed under the 'umbrella' nomenclature of critical care. The development of such units has also emphasised the need for a trained nurses in this specialist area (Lassen 1953). This required provision of specialised post-registration courses for nurses, and has resulted in several professional organisations and journals specifically addressing critical care nursing issues.

In today's health system, intensive care is seen at one end of a spectrum of acute care, with ward care providing the opposite end of the spectrum. High dependency units provide the intermediate level of care between the two, although the provision of such units remains a contentious issue (Edbrookes 1996). Intensive care units provide comprehensive support for patients with immediate life threatening crises, and support for their families and friends. With an emphasis on medical need and availability of technology, intensive care units offer potentially life saving interventions during acute physiological crises (Intensive Care Society 1990). Intensive care provides:

> a service for patients with potentially recoverable conditions who can benefit from more detailed observation and invasive treatment than can safely be provided in general wards or high dependency areas.
>
> (DoH 1996a, p. 6)

In the UK, intensive care is a costly and labour intensive resource, accounting for 1 per cent of the total acute care hospital beds (Dorman 1996). The UK spends an estimated £675 million per year on intensive care (Edbrookes *et al.* 1997) representing approximately 2 per cent of the hospital budget. The nursing budget accounts for 75 per cent of the intensive care expenditure due to the high nurse–patient ratio required within these units (DoH 1996a). Patient admission to intensive care reflects both demographic patterns and the hospital population as a whole. Patients cared for in these units are therefore increasingly older and present with acute exacerbation of long-term chronic disease (Dragsted and Qvist 1992). This is reflected in an unpredictable patient outcome. Recent data demonstrates that 15–35 per cent of patients die during intensive care treatment (Audit Commission 1999).

As technology continues to develop, there is an ever increasing demand on intensive care facilities. In contrast to the large critical care facilities in America (Seymour 2001), intensive care units in the UK remain much smaller with on average six beds. Recent audit has demonstrated that although the availability of intensive care is unevenly spread across the country, nine out of ten acute NHS trusts now have some form of intensive care unit (Audit Commission 1999). Indeed, intensive care has become a routine part of the post-operative management of the more complex surgical procedures (Crosby and Rees 1994). Intensive care is seen to influence practices and treatments across acute care. Treatment and procedures once limited to intensive care have since become integrated into ordinary practices within the hospital organisation (Seymour *op. cit.*).

Intensive care has recently received a high national profile as demand on intensive care beds has exceeded supply, resulting in wide coverage in the national press (Daily Telegraph 2000). Additionally, a shortage in specially educated intensive care nurses has led, in some units, to the closure of intensive care beds (Rennie 1999). These events have occurred against a backdrop of growing pressure on ward staff to manage increasingly sicker patients, at the same time as striving to

meet government waiting list targets. This has directly impacted on the intensive care workload and throughput. Intensive care units continue to expand,
consuming vast financial and human resources, despite the lack of outcome
measurements of these speciality units (Zussman 1992). There is evidence to
suggest these issues are also reflected in the provision of intensive care inter-
nationally (Brilli et al. 2001).

Current workforce constraints within the NHS have reflected on the
availability of trained medical and non-medical personnel to work in intensive
care. To meet the need for specialised training in Intensive Care Medicine,
recommendations have been made by the Intercollegiate Board for Training
in Intensive Care Medicine. These proposals advocate that medical students,
doctors in acute hospital specialities and those wishing to pursue a full-time
career in this speciality all receive a structured exposure to this clinical area.
Although these recommendations have substantial advantages for the delivery
of health care (Smith 1998a), educational support and resource is required
to meet the curricula demands of such programmes. This not only requires
senior medical staff to be committed to education and training, but also places
increasing demands on nursing staff to support junior medical staff in the
principles of managing critically ill patients (Webb 1996).

Therefore, while intensive care is often seen as a medically driven speciality 'it
should be recognised that all members of the multidisciplinary team are crucial
to patient care and outcome' (Smith 1998b, p. 115). Intensive care is therefore
optimally delivered to the patient by a team of highly trained personnel.
Supported by technicians, managers and accountants, this team comprises
pharmacists, physiotherapists, dieticians, and the doctors and nurses in the
intensive care unit.

The nursing role in intensive care

As discussed earlier, health care advances required response from all health care
personnel to develop their practice base. Intensive care was, and continues to
be, exposed to a significant increase in the use of technology as a result of developments in medical science. This has presented a conflict for nurses in balancing
the science of technology with the art of nursing (Henderson 1980; Ashworth
1990).

Noc and Weil (1996) both intensive care consultants, identified the key
nursing responsibilities to be aligned with the science of technology through
involvement with maintaining patient observations and the responsibility for
gathering all non-invasive and invasive laboratory data. Through this focus on
technical functions undertaken by nurses in intensive care, intensive care nursing
becomes solely defined by the medical care required to deliver the service
(Fairman 1992).

The emphasis on nursing delivering medical care has been challenged with
appeals for nursing to preserve humanity in an age of technology (Mann 1992).

Woodrow (1997) argues that despite the fact that clinical practice is focused on multiple system failure support, this provides but one challenge for the nurse clinician who chooses to work in the intensive care environment. Intensive care nurses are seen to provide the link between the patient and machine. In this way, not only is technological competence demonstrated, but also compassion and the humanitarian aspects of nursing. This is further supported through the empirical work of Chenitz and Swanson (1986), Benner (1984), and Anspach (1993).

This debate continues to dominate pre-occupations with developing roles today. Thirty years ago the different practices of medicine and nursing in intensive care were easily identifiable (Roth and Daze 1984). This distinction was based on the intensive care nurse initiating treatment based on the assessment of the patient's symptoms, and not through making differential medical diagnosis. The contemporary role of the intensive care nurse has since developed with the addition of tasks from medicine (role extension) and the development of nursing (role expansion) through enhanced nursing knowledge and skills (Hunt and Wainwright 1994).

Whilst the boundary between contemporary nursing and medicine in intensive care is arguably unclear (Webb 1996), it is apparent the nursing role is developing skills and knowledge that was once perceived to be the sole domain of medicine. Examples of this include increased involvement and responsibility with patient weaning from the ventilator (Anderson and O'Brien 1995) and drug and fluid prescription (DoH 1996a).

To further explore nursing role developments and nurse led clinical decision making in intensive care, the Royal College of Nursing (1997) undertook a telephone survey of eighty-nine intensive care units. The results demonstrated that the intensive care nurses surveyed were experiencing considerable role change associated with increased workload and responsibility. The driving forces for this were identified to be within the nursing profession itself, and driven by external forces, e.g. junior doctors' hours (DoH 1991). Intensive care nurses were 'equal to the challenge of a more advanced medical and technological care whilst retaining a strong sense of the value of nursing care to patients and families' (Royal College of Nursing 1997, p. 9). Similar international trends about the nature of nursing in the intensive care setting have been demonstrated (Street 1992; Chamberliss 1996).

Jowett (1986) described the intensive care nurse as the key to successful patient management. In this clinical area, nurses are perceived as achieving greater autonomy and enjoying good working relationships with medical colleagues (Baggs and Ryan 1990). Despite the general nursing recruitment problems, intensive care remains one of the more appealing areas of the health service for nurses (Ball 1997). The prospect of working one to one with a patient and family for a whole shift is a key attraction for nursing staff. In addition, a large percentage of nurses are educationally prepared and supported to work in this speciality to diploma or degree level (Audit Commission 1999). An appropriately qualified intensive care nurse therefore has: 'an appropriate knowledge base in adult critical care, high level decision making skills and sensitivity to the needs of the critically ill and those close to them' (Ball 2001, p. 5).

In summary, intensive care has been identified as a highly complex area with high levels of uncertainty and instability above other hospital care areas (Leatt and Schneck 1981). Despite the fact that there have undoubtedly been changes in the acuity of all care areas since this observation was made, the intensive care environment continues to be unpredictable and complex. It is this level of complexity and responsiveness to need that has driven the roles required within the intensive care environment.

What is evident from this discussion is that the context of care defines the nature of health care roles, and of the health care team. In primary care, the nursing practice role is described as independent practice with interdisciplinary consultation and referral (DeAngelis 1994). As highlighted by Brilli et al. (2001), many disciplines work together in critical care to meet complex patient needs. The nature of care provided to critically ill patients requires team working that is built on foundations of interdependent practice (Hickey et al. 1996).

The intensive care environment, and the medical and nursing roles within it, are used here as a case for analysis. In some ways, intensive care is presented as the extreme of a case: a clinical area that, as the following chapters will reveal, represents a highly acute yet controlled environment that challenges definitions of what medical and nursing roles actually constitute. In other ways, there are recurring themes that resonate across health care areas. In this book, I am not making the assertion that the findings from this work are directly transferable to other clinical settings. It is for the reader to make that supposition in an informed and critical manner, cognisant of their own work culture, and of the local existence of the ideals and political interests (Hammersley 1993).

Chapter 2

Collaboration
Working partnerships or sleeping with the enemy?

The previous chapter has explored the contextual issues that have influenced medical and nursing roles. This chapter has, as its focus, how doctors and nurses work together in the clinical environment. Review of the literature demonstrates that much has been written on the nature of working relationships between doctors and nurses. In this section, I will critically review the concepts that most frequently arise in literature relating to doctor–nurse relationships. The terms used to describe clinical team functioning are explored, together with the specific concept of collaboration. As the review will demonstrate, over time there have been subtle changes in the definitions used to describe team working. I suggest that these reflect the historical socialisation and contemporary dynamics of health care teams. Such definitions and developments, therefore, need to be understood cognisant of the health care context at that time.

In the latter half of this chapter, I explore the nursing and sociological literature to examine interdisciplinary working in order to understand the working relationships between doctors and nurses. This review will demonstrate how sociological perspectives can provide alternative readings on everyday clinical events, such as the ward round and the nursing handover. The chapter concludes with consideration of whether collaborative working partnerships are of interest to all within the health care team.

Collaboration in health care: definitions and concepts

- Many frameworks and concepts have been used to describe the working relationships between medicine and nursing. At present, the most frequently cited concept in health care policy and literature is that of 'collaboration', meaning 'to labour together': although alternative definitions are offered that imply a willingness to co-operate with one's enemy (Webster 1990).

Collaboration is defined as being non-hierarchical in nature and a 'co-operative venture based on shared power and authority. It assumes power based on a knowledge base or expertise as opposed to power shared on role or function'

(Knaus 1980, p. 12). The principle of joint decision making, whilst respecting the unique qualities and abilities of each professional (Coluccio and Maguire 1983), is paramount in collaborative relationships. Leathard (1994) provides a useful taxonomy offering some structure to the many terms currently used to describe team working:

- *Concept based*: team work, collaboration, co-ordination, integration
- *Agency based*: interagency, intersectorial, multi-professional
- *Process based*: co-operative, collegial, working together
- *Outcome based*: shared governance
- *Power based*: interdependency

As our understanding of the historical socialisation of the disciplines and the changing interactions between professions develops, terms used to describe how health care teams work are refined (McCallin 2001). Several years ago, most health care professionals, including myself, used to refer to 'multidisciplinary working' and 'multidisciplinary teams'. 'Multidisciplinary' is now used to describe a team process where members of different disciplines manage patients independently, then share information with each other. The more popularly espoused term 'interdisciplinary' alludes to a level of collaboration requiring joint development of a plan of care with professionals pooling their knowledge (Sorrells-Jones 1997). Through this, there is greater emphasis on collection action and process orientation. Although the changing perspectives may reflect the importance placed by society on the integration of tasks, there continues to be a problem in achieving a consensus definition on collaboration.

Through enhancing quality of care, collaboration is accredited with improving patient outcomes that could not be achieved if health care practices were organised differently. Patient needs are placed paramount, with collaboration providing a synergistic alliance that optimises the contribution of each participant (Weiss and Davis 1985). Collaboration is fundamentally a relationship, with many of the elements of collaborative working being vital in any partnership (Miccolo and Spanier 1993) and requires co-operation; common goals and co-ordination of activities; and interdependence and mutual respect (Neubauer 1993). Collaborative practice is a dynamic process requiring time, energy, and commitment (Makaram 1995). This will necessitate a radical culture change in a health care climate of uncertainty, suspicion, and competition (Fatchett 1996). Collaboration is concerned with organisational and practitioner culture (Trevillion 1995), and acknowledges growing interdependence amongst health care professionals (King 1990).

The promotion of collaboration remains an important theme and continues to underpin current UK health policy. It is one of the key principles embedded in the changes proposed in the Government White Paper '*The New NHS: Modern, Dependable*':

to be a success then there is a need for the National Health Service to work in partnership, to break down organisational barriers, to forge stronger links and to put the needs of the patients at the centre of the process.

(DoH 1997, 2.4)

As a buzzword of the 1990s, the term 'collaboration' can be found woven throughout both academic and policy texts, including Leathard (1994) and (DoH 1999, 2000b). There is a continued interest and focus on professional working relationships within the health care team. The key drivers for this relate to the perceived need to rationalise services and the provision of a more effective, integrated service, for users and professions (Ovretveit *et al.* 1997).

Despite the vast amount of literature focusing on collaboration, the lack of a consensus definition on collaboration makes concept analysis in empirical work problematic (Taylor 1996). The identification of antecedents, consequences and empirical referents is reliant on rhetoric, rather than empirical research (Hennemann 1995) and evaluation of the effectiveness of collaboration is there- fore problematic. In acknowledging these limitations, the studies that have been undertaken on collaborative doctor–nurse relationships will now be explored. To provide structure to this, I will explore the health care literature first, followed with sociological perspectives.

Collaboration: health care perspectives

There is much discussion in the nursing literature about the nature of doctor– nurse relationships, but the empirical base for this area is poorly developed (Ross and Mackenzie 1996). The majority of the studies undertaken in this research area are North American, provoking caution in generalising the results. Much of the UK literature remains mainly anecdotal, and rarely analytical. Tables 2.1 and 2.2 provide outlines of the main literature related to medical and nursing collaboration and outcome evaluation. The tables have been developed through review of the collaborative literature with identification of key patient, provider (medical and nursing) and organisational outcomes. These tables demonstrate that the body of the literature specifically highlights the outcomes for the providers of care, with nurses having a high concern, and regard, for collaboration.

Although the majority of the literature on collaboration is based on opinion and rhetoric, there are key seminal empirical works that have influenced our understanding of collaboration. I will now explore these in some depth. The work of the most influential contributors, the North American nurse researchers, Sandra Weiss and Judith Baggs, will be given specific consideration.

Many of the early writers based their definition of collaboration on a model conceptualised by Rubel and Thomas (1976). This work was specifically related to conflict management; an interesting application in itself. Within this model, collaboration was seen to combine a high level of co-operation and concern for others, with assertiveness requiring a concern for self.

Table 2.1 Outcomes of collaboration matrix

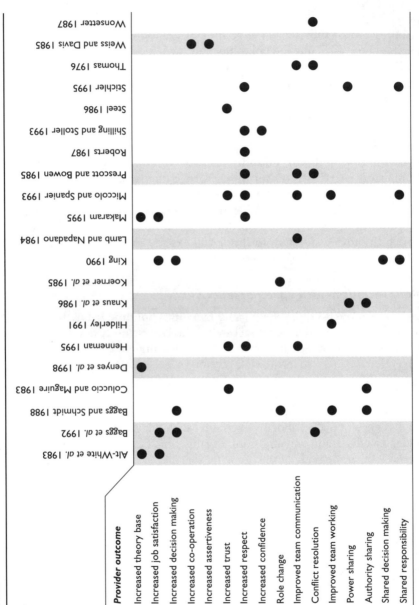

Source: Research

Source: Opinion Paper

Table 2.2 Outcomes of collaboration matrix

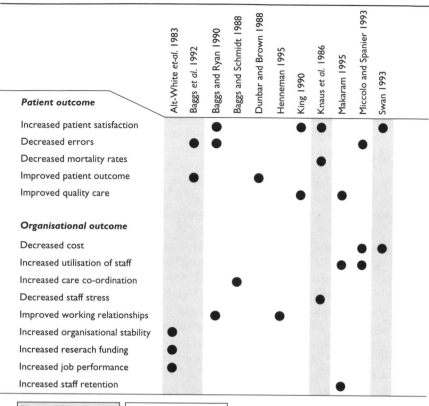

	Alt-White et al. 1983	Baggs et al. 1992	Baggs and Ryan 1990	Baggs and Schmidt 1988	Dunbar and Brown 1988	Henneman 1995	King 1990	Knaus et al. 1986	Makaram 1995	Miccolo and Spanier 1993	Swan 1993
Patient outcome											
Increased patient satisfaction			●				●	●			●
Decreased errors		●	●						●		
Decreased mortality rates								●			
Improved patient outcome		●			●						
Improved quality care							●	●			
Organisational outcome											
Decreased cost										●	●
Increased utilisation of staff									●	●	
Increased care co-ordination				●							
Decreased staff stress								●			
Improved working relationships			●			●					
Increased organisational stability	●										
Increased reserach funding	●										
Increased job performance	●										
Increased staff retention									●		

Source: Research		Source: Opinion Paper

Weiss (1983) developed this model to explore the wider aspects of inter-personal relationships in health care. In conjunction with unstructured interviews with nurses, doctors and patients, two collaborative practice measurement scales (one for doctors, one for nurses) were developed. Weiss's (1983) paper was one of the earliest to empirically explore the concept of collaboration within a health care setting. The collaborative practice scales (CPS) were further developed and, were finally tested with Weiss and Davis (1985). The CPS was structured through use of Likert-type statements to measure specific features of collaboration. For example, this included the question 'I consider nurses' opinions when developing a treatment plan' (Weiss and Davis 1985, p. 300).

The results on the validity and reliability of the scales were reported in 1985 (Weiss and Davis *op. cit.*). Initially a random sample of 200 doctors and 200 nurses were selected to test the scales. Due to a poor medical staff response rate (response rate: nurses 47.5 per cent, doctors 21.5 per cent), a further 200 medical staff were recruited, finally giving a total sample of 94 doctors. The cause of the poor response rate of the medical staff was not explored. Although the scales were said to demonstrate reliability, the conclusions were non-specific. Despite the apparent limited development of Thomas's original theory, Weiss's paper was hailed as new and influential (Jones 1994). This study explored only two variables related to collaboration: assertiveness and co-operation, and other potential influences, including autonomy of roles, role definition and communication were not acknowledged.

In a multi-method research study by Knaus *et al.* (1986), the treatment and outcome of patients in thirteen American intensive care units were compared. A total of 5,030 patients were studied through comparison of data on pre-treatment risk of death using a validated scale (Acute Physiology and Chronic Health Evaluation II) and the actual mortality rate. Unit profiles were also obtained through questionnaires completed by medical or nursing directors. These profiles demonstrated that there were similar technical and support capabilities across the units, but that organisational, staffing, research and educational differences existed.

Knaus's study (*op. cit.*) demonstrated that important differences between the predicted and observed patient mortality rates appeared to be related to the interaction and communication between doctors and nurses. Despite the fact that the findings of this work are often quoted in the professional literature, there are some limitations that require highlighting. Apart from the concern of self-reporting used in the unit profile as a data collection strategy, there are other data collection issues. In determining the predicted and actual patient mortality rates, the only other key variables explored related to organisational and educational areas. There was no data collection regarding pre-admission, treatment or discharge facilities, which could influence patient outcome.

There was no reference to the admission criteria of the units. If units admitted less dependent patients for monitoring only, this could have dramatically influenced the mortality rates and patient outcomes in those units. Case mix adjustment was not, at that time developed.

Stimulated by Knaus's work, Baggs and Schmitt (1988) undertook an extensive literature review into collaboration and identified four critical attributes of collaboration: shared responsibility for planning; shared decision making; open communication; and co-ordination of care. From this review, both patient and nurse advantages were identified highlighting beneficial outcomes including reduced patient costs, increased organisational efficiency, and reduced team stress.

Baggs *et al.* (1992) further developed this work to explore the association between interdisciplinary collaboration and patient outcomes. In order to explore this more fully, the specific area of patient transfer was identified. Questionnaires were administered to 56 nurses and 31 doctors on a medical intensive care unit during 286 consecutive patient transfers. Three questionnaires were used: decision about transfer scale (DATS), Weiss and Davis' collaborative practice scale (CPS) and the Index of Work Satisfaction (IWS). The IWS was only administered to nurses.

The results revealed that doctors and nurses scored similarly for satisfaction, but differently on collaboration. This led to the conclusion that collaboration was strongly linked to satisfaction for nurses, but was weakly linked for doctors. Although this was a rigorous study and issues of reliability and validity were addressed, no definitive results were presented. However, this is one of the many research papers to intimate that doctors and nurses may have different perceptions, definitions and expectations of collaboration.

This different understanding and expectations that health care professionals have regarding collaboration was reflected in Prescott and Bowen's (1985) North American work. In this, a national survey of 536 doctors and 264 nurses was undertaken, together with interviews from 180 doctors and 264 nurses in 15 metropolitan hospitals. The results demonstrated that respondents reported satisfactory working relationships, but used different definitions for nurse–doctor relationships. Nurses emphasised mutual respect and trust where doctors used nurse communication with the medical staff, nurses' willingness to help and nurse competence as key indicators to a satisfactory working relationship.

The concept of collaborative working was further developed through Baggs's 1994 work to develop an instrument to measure collaboration and satisfaction about care transfer decisions. The tool was tested (Baggs et al. 1997) in three critical care units, using a total of 1,432 patient transfers. Patients who had limitations placed on their treatment were not used in this study. As ethical decision making, including medical decisions on patient treatment limitations is a noted source of concern for nurses (Grundstein-Amado 1992; Robertson 1996; Viney 1996), this work did ignore a key area that may impact on collaborative practices between medical and nursing staff. Baggs et al. (op. cit.) used two measurement scales to determine collaboration and satisfaction between nurses and doctors: the collaboration and satisfaction regarding care decisions and the Index of Work Satisfaction, which was again only administered to nurses. Although nurses and doctors reported moderate amounts of collaboration, it was the nursing staff that reported reduced satisfaction with decision making in comparison to the medical staff.

Baggs's interest in collaboration has continued with publication in 1999 of a study to investigate the association of collaboration between ICU doctors and nurses and patient outcomes. When patients were ready for transfer from the ICU, questionnaires were again issued to staff to assess care providers' reports of collaboration. After controlling for severity of illness, the association between interprofessional collaboration and patient outcome was assessed. This was a large study using 1,432 patient discharges. The results demonstrated that there were improved patient outcomes associated with nurses reporting greater collaboration between medical and nursing teams, but there was no association with doctor-reported levels of collaboration. This again lends tentative weight to collaboration being of importance to nurses, and the impact that this may have on patient outcome.

This review of key health care studies on collaboration has not only highlighted the different medical and nursing interpretation on collaboration, but emphasised the lack of medical curiosity in this area. From the above studies, Knaus (*op. cit.*) was the only work undertaken by a doctor. Until recently, little had been published in the medical literature about collaborative relationships within the clinical team, or about working relationships with nursing *per se*. The traditional medical response to the development of collaborative partnerships in health care has tended to elicit concerns regarding encroachment on medical territory or authority (Payne 1999). Nevertheless, recent medical practice (Robotham 1999), medical policy (General Medical Council 1995), and medical publishing (Davies *et al.* 1999) have all demonstrated an increasing appreciation of the need for positive doctor–nurse relationships.

The key studies outlined above predominantly relate to collaboration and team satisfaction. The effect of doctor–nurse collaboration on patients is not well addressed. Despite this lack of outcome based work, health care practitioners are required to collaborate in order to provide flexible responses to health care need (DoH 1996b, 1999, 2000b). Modern health care relies increasingly on teamwork through the development of interprofessional teams. These teams are located not only within the hospital and primary care settings, but across the traditional boundaries of health and social care.

A health care philosophy based on interdependence and mutual respect may be difficult to be realised in practice. Research has demonstrated that nurses have been dissatisfied with their working relationship with medicine over the past century (Pilliteri and Ackerman 1993). A survey conducted with British and Australian nurses (Adamson *et al.* 1995) revealed that nurses from both countries remain dissatisfied with many aspects of their working conditions, including their relationships with medical staff. Indeed, satisfaction with working relationships with medical and management staff were key in nurses defining a good intensive care unit (Darvas and Hawkins 2002).

It is interesting that the joint initiative between the *Nursing Times* and *British Medical Journal* on working relationships between doctors and nurses (Salvage and Smith 2000) prompted such a diverse range of responses. In the latter publication, it was demonstrated that nurses and doctors can safely and effectively adjust their working boundaries for patient benefit. Nonetheless, there were still assertions being made that medicine was still too slow to adjust; that nursing was sacrificing its best attributes; and that there was a need for a stronger empirical base for collaboration before medicine would change. As Salvage and Smith comment: 'the core dynamic is the same: nursing, for all its new independence and expertise, is still dancing around the medical maypole' (Salvage and Smith 2000, p. 1019).

The review of the nursing literature to date has demonstrated that the nature of doctor–nurse working relationships is an area of concern, but predominantly to nurses. Within this, the concept of collaboration holds a central position. Although both medicine and nursing value team working, different values and descriptors are used. Stein (1967) remarked that the doctor–nurse relationship led to competition, conflict, and distorted communication. Such conflict is multifaceted and deeply woven in a mesh of economic, social and professional issues (Alpert 1992).

• Doctor–nurse relationships: sociological perspectives

Interprofessional conflicts have been documented since the time of Florence Nightingale (Kalisch and Kalisch 1977). Therefore understanding these conflicts requires a comprehension of the historical traditions of both professions, the traditional gender relationships, and the hierarchical nature of health care organisations. In normative terms, nursing and medicine reflects two different cultures with contradictory visions (Temkin-Greener 1983). In this, medicine emphasises the status quo of its traditional authority, within an inherently hierarchical organisation and function. Nursing, however, stresses a more egalitarian vision of power relations with collaboration and peer co-operation as prerequisites for team care provision (Prescott and Bowen 1985).

Key studies for understanding professionals and their interactions have historically relied on such work as Freidson (1970) and Stein (1967). The thrust of these works have argued that doctors hold a dominant and unchallenged position in health care, by virtue of their knowledge base and their societal position (Freidson 1970). This has led to interplay between doctors and nurses, referred to as playing the game (Stein 1967). The problem, as identified by Stein, was a lack of communication and assertion by nurses.

Stein later re-visited this topic (Stein et al. 1990) identifying societal trends as being the main instigators of the problem, and that nurses no longer wanted to 'play the game'. The solution was again put forward that nurses needed to become more assertive. What this approach did not address was the fundamental structural problem of the hierarchy between nursing and medicine. Stein's study has been highly influential in the area of the doctor–nurse relationship, but it must be recognised that his original work was not based on an extensive research process.

Empirical studies have since challenged Stein's rules of 'the game'. In Hughes's (1988) participant observational study of casualty work in a British unit, three situational factors were identified which acted to promote the power of nurses in the study: the complex workload; high medical turnover; and high proportion of doctors from the Asian subcontinent which led to greater nursing influence in the unit. Porter (1998) has since given a more contemporary and critical interpretation of these findings.

With an interest in how power relations are manifest between nurses and doctors, Porter (1991) undertook a participant observational study on an intensive care unit in Northern Ireland. The results demonstrated that nurses did possess and utilise considerable power in patient care decisions through an informal but covert decision-making style. Evidence of formal overt decision-making was limited. Porter argued that these results demonstrated that there had indeed been historical progression in patient care decision making. He suggested that a more overt style of decision making would only be achieved through achieving greater diagnostic autonomy, for example, through reformulation of the nursing process. This work is complemented by Porter's (1995) later critical realist ethnography that furthers understanding of nursing's relationship with medicine through analysing participant observational data obtained from medical and intensive care areas.

In order to explore the issue of autonomy and professional authority, Walby and Greenwall's (1994) work focused on medical and nursing negotiation of interprofessional boundaries. Data from interviews with doctors and nurses in five English hospitals were used. The historical functions of care and treatment were areas used to distinguish between medical and nursing work. Key areas of contested authority were related to the control of patient treatment, task priorities and nurse–manager–doctor conflict. The authority of the consultant was seen as paramount in patient management; in setting of practice guidelines; and through influence on nursing management issues. Through this, the historical and symbolic hierarchical relationship of medicine over nursing was then reinforced.

Svensson (1996) explored doctor–nurse interplay using a negotiated order perspective that upholds all social orders to be negotiated (Strauss 1978). This was considered to provide a more flexible approach to study professional inter-actions than the traditional authoritarian model proposed by Freidson (1970). Svensson (op. cit.) interviewed 45 nurses from 14 wards in 5 Swedish hospitals. Analysis of the transcripts revealed that a strong nursing voice was presented in the nursing interviews. In identifying the social needs of the patient and co-ordinating care, nurses felt themselves to be in a unique position. When discussing patient treatment issues within the medical treatment domain, there was still some evidence of Stein's (op. cit.) game being played. Although this work developed the use of a negotiated order perspective in nursing research, it has some limitations. As the study was located in a non-critical care area in Sweden, caution must be exercised on generalising the results.

The concept of negotiated order was further developed by Allen (1997, 2001) through an ethnographic study on the occupational jurisdiction of nurses. This was achieved through fieldwork undertaken on a medical and surgical ward in a single United Kingdom trust. In addition, 57 doctors, nurses and managers within those areas were also interviewed. The aim of the research was to undertake analysis of the negotiation process in the workplace, with particular attention to the members' talk. Allen's results demonstrated that there were changing role boundaries and changing divisions of labour.

In Allen's work (op. cit.) there were many examples of contested inter-professional boundaries, but little evidence of inter-occupational conflict and negotiations. The conclusion drawn by Allen was that nurses personally manage the boundaries of their work, thereby minimising conflict. Similar to the results found in Hughes's work (1988), temporal-spatial organisation of care work were seen to be an important issue for managing roles and the division of labour. Allen suggested that nurses developed strategies to manage the tensions associated with the social organisation of hospital work that were non-negotiated, and that this informal boundary blurring was a 'taken for granted' feature of nursing practice.

Wicks (1995) explored this characteristic in her paper on 'Nurses and doctors and discourses of healing'. In this ethnographic study, based in an Australian hospital, Wicks used post-structuralist theory to re-introduce the notion of agency into analysis of nursing work. The dichotomous relationship between care and cure was once more highlighted, but rather than attempting to 'play the game', nurses were seen to use power contained within nursing knowledge to overcome the established power differentials.

As this brief overview of the key sociological works has shown, a substantial paradigmatic and pragmatic shift has occurred in the conceptualisation of the nursing role within doctor–nurse relationships. Whilst the initial theory development was influenced by the deterministic work of Freidson in the 1970s, the more recent contemporary work has been influenced by post-structuralist and feminist thought. A key practice change identified within the recent studies suggests that nursing is beginning to manage the division of labour and to shift the power base within the team-working relationships. To explore this area further, I will now present a more specific review on health care team relationships and patient care decision making.

The ward round and the health care team: sociological perspectives

In the sociological literature concerning doctor–nurse relationships and patient care decisions, one specific forum provides the main focus: the ward round. Decisions regarding patient care can occur at any time of the patient's stay, and the ward round is one of the clinical forums that brings together the entire health care team involved in patient care. In recent years, this has become a strong focus for sociological study in order to understand the complex processes involved in health care team working. Sociological studies focusing on the involvement of the health care team in the ward round will now be reviewed.

From a sociological perspective, the ward round is seen as an example of ritual, an important feature in any society (Helman 1990), which re-states the values and rules that bring group coherence, and manages group uncertainties. Turner (1986) asserts that rituals symbolically portray key values; this then enables cultural orientations to be understood in context. The ward round, as ritual, is explored by Walsh and Ford (1989). Within their analysis, the ward round is seen to have several purposes including assisting in the continuity of care and information transfer. As the following section will demonstrate, this clinical decision-making forum has been frequently used in order to explore dynamics within the health care team.

Busby and Gilchrist's (1992) observational study was driven by perceived communication inadequacies in UK health care. The ward round was chosen as the focus of the study due to its many discourses. During the several weeks observation period, the daily ward rounds of three medical consultants were observed, that included 21 nurses and 19 patients. Data were collected through use of an observation schedule that was used to code all verbal behaviours. Further data were collected though interviews with 8 of the patients and questionnaires that were sent to 60 staff. Although Busby and Gilchrist (*op. cit.*) document a well-conducted study, it is not made clear whether only consultants were observed or if all the medical team were included in the observational component of the study. In addition, it is important to stress that only verbal behaviours were used to measure communication in this study.

The study findings demonstrated that nurses perceived their main ward round role to be information giving, patient advocacy, and asking questions on behalf of the patients. Although consultants identified that nurses had a high knowledge of the patients, consultants asked the junior doctor for details regarding the patient 67 per cent of the time. Analysis of the 2,391 observed interactions demonstrated that only 12 per cent of comments were made by, and only 10 per cent of discussion directed at, nurses. Nurses were only asked their opinion four times throughout the duration of the study. The majority of the discussion with nurses was related to patient symptom and treatment, only 12 per cent of the comments were related to social matters or focused on emotional or psychological matters. Whilst from the content analysis of the interviews, the nurses perceived themselves to be assertive in the ward round, analysis of the observational part of the study, demonstrated a lack of assertive behaviour by the nurses.

Nearly a decade after Busby and Gilchrist's work (*op. cit.*), similar themes continue to arise. In Manias and Street's (2001b) critical ethnographic study, the participation of critical care nurses in ward round was explored. Using data collection methods of professional journaling, participant observation and interviews, six nurses participated in the study. The findings demonstrated that nursing remains marginalised in the ward rounds, confined to supplementing information and providing further information about patient assessment to medical staff. The concept of 'contesting spaces' was used to explore how nurses, despite tremendous difficulties, were taking the opportunity to participate in the decision-making process in the ward round.

Using a post-modernist analysis in his ethnographic research, Fox (1993) documented social processes that occurred during surgical ward rounds at two general hospitals. Despite the fact that the focus of this research concerned the definition of surgery by the doctor and the patient, it has some significant theoretical and methodological pointers. In Fox's work, it was suggested that interactions between the doctor and patient could be viewed as a meeting between experts, one possessing authoritative knowledge by virtue of professional education, the other through ownership of the body itself (Tuckett *et al.* 1985).

Fox's study used power and authority as its focus and examined how surgeons manipulated ward round interactions to sustain their perceptions of surgery and healing. It identified ward rounds as an organisational strategy used by surgeons to achieve discursive hegemony. This was achieved through maintaining control over the content and pattern of the dialogue within the ward round. Analysis of the observational data revealed three surgeon-centred themes: the discourse on patient physiology, the discourse on wound condition, and the discourse on recovery and discharge. The conclusion drawn was that the ward round was a tightly controlled occupational strategy. Through this, the surgeons maintained their authority due to the power of the organisational interactions.

Through such studies, it is clear that the ward round is a powerful ritual within health care. The ward round is a forum where analysis of the interplay between health care staff and patients demonstrates competing discourses. The interplay of these discourses reveals situations where the dominant players act out influence and authority.

The assertion of the nursing voice has been further explored in several studies. The concept of deputed medical power is explored in Parker and Wiltshire's (1995) study of nursing handover in a major metropolitan hospital in Australia and in Ekman and Segestein's (1995) ethnographic study on a Swedish medical ward. Deputed medical power was used to describe the continued evidence of medical control over nursing work. Although the nursing handover was the focus for both these studies, similar themes as documented throughout this chapter, emerge. Both were relatively small studies with the data sources being the oral handover and written patient progress notes. From the key emerging themes, the nursing voice was perceived as weak, and often an echo of the medical voice. This silence was linked to powerful hegemonic forces of medicine, considered to be the dominant discourse within the health care system.

For me, these final papers highlight some interesting issues. A key stance inferred by them was that medical and nursing work is polarised. I offer a more moderated position. Even though I can acknowledge the distinctness of medicine and nursing in my own area of practice, I can also recognise areas of similarity: I do not think that we can shy away from the reality of this. For me, the issue is not only about the uniqueness of role and function, but also the realisation that there are some intrinsic similarities. It is how the roles and the work undertaken contributes to patient focused care that is most important.

Concluding thoughts

These first two chapters have demonstrated how health care developments have caused role boundaries between nursing and medicine to become unclear: 'What today are essential medical tasks will change over time as technology progresses' (DoH 1991, p. 226). Due to the nature of contemporary health care and the requisite responsibilities, roles are becoming blurred, and this is particularly so for nursing.

One of the key issues to arise from the policy and professional literature relates to the recognition of complementary roles in order to understand working relationships, and has been described as mutual interdependence (Fagin 1992). This reflects personal beliefs that nursing and medicine are inextricably linked. There is a mutual dependency, which requires effective working patterns to be adopted by all. As observed by Stein *et al.* in the 1990 re-visiting of 'The doctor nurse game':

> Physicians [doctors] and nurses can both benefit if their relationship becomes more mutually interdependent. Subservient and dominant roles are both psychologically restricting. When a subordinate becomes liberated, there is the potential for the dominant one to become liberated too.
>
> (Stein *et al.* 1990, p. 549)

It is clear that there is considerable interest in how clinical teams work, with nurses demonstrating a substantial clinical and empirical interest in this area. This nursing concern is also reflected in national policy documents (DoH 1997, DoH 2000b, DoH 2001a), and receives particular emphasis in the national nursing strategy document (DoH 1999). In this, it is maintained that in order for nurses to enhance the contribution to the health team and provide improved patient care, greater attention will need to be focused on the design of team and role boundaries (DoH 1999).

As identified by Blue and Fitzgerald (2002), this degree of nursing attention may result from nurses holding the curiosity and research expertise required to explore this fundamentally sociological area. An alternative explanation to the high level of nursing activity in this area could be the indifference demonstrated by medical staff about team working relationships. If there is even an element of truth in the latter option, then in order to re-define new teams to meet service and patient need, this will indeed require a significant shift in organisational culture, and the commitment from all clinical staff.

Chapter 3

Clinical management teams
The impact of general management

Previous chapters have explored the clinical role of the nurse and mapped working relationships between doctors and nurses through exposition of developments in clinical working environments. The clinical domain is but one arena in which nursing and medical staff interact. This chapter explores another area within which medicine and nursing operates, that of the service domain of health care practice. The term 'service domain' is used to describe any area relating to the management of clinical units, and of the clinical service. Such activity occurs not at the micro patient interface level, but at middle management level or the clinical unit–trust interface. At its most influential, this area can then extend to involvement in executive and national policy level decisions. It requires nurses, doctors and health service managers to make operational and strategic decisions about the delivery of the service, rather than be directly involved with patient management. This, therefore, offers a comparative area to explore the working relationships between doctors and nurses, who both work with managers in order to deliver the clinical service.

In order to understand the nursing role in the service domain, I begin this chapter with a review of the introduction of management structures into the NHS. I particularly focus on service changes that have occurred since the 1970s. This chapter simply describes the impact of the health policy initiatives and the resultant management structure changes on the nursing role. I do not set out to explore, nor to ignore, the presence of management discourses that can be located within nursing, nor the clinical values that underpin the principles of managers (Traynor 1999).

The introduction of general management principles into the health service has raised important issues about health care professionals working within a managerial structure. This area is explored through discussion of working relationships between managers and health care professionals at local clinical unit level. The consequences of the NHS re-organisations at this level are explored, and the implications for those involved in health care management are examined. Through this, I will demonstrate that the ways that clinical management teams have developed, and the evolution of roles within these teams, have similar tensions to the clinical practice domain.

In the concluding section of this chapter, I focus on nurses' ability to influence decision making in the wider health policy context. Once again, the key challenges for nursing that have been explored in the scene setting chapters will resonate through. The prevailing roles that medicine and nursing hold in decision making across the health care spectrum will be made explicit.

The introduction of general management into the health service

At the start of the NHS, a diplomacy model of management existed where the role of the manager enabled health care professionals to care for the patient. Medical staff were highly influential and powerful in determining the shape of the service, whilst managers were reactive and focused on managing internal organisational issues (Harrison et al. 1992).

In the 1970s, the political and economic climate began to shift. There was increasing public and governmental unease over rising costs, marked financial constraints, and resourcing problems (Elston 1991). The contribution of high technology medicine was questioned (McKeown 1976) which, together with the more radical claims of epidemic iatrogenesis (Illich 1977), created a climate for political questioning of the effectiveness and efficiency of medicine.

At that time, the NHS functioned following a relatively simple model. In a pyramidal structure, policy and control flowed down from the government via the DoH, to increasingly smaller geographical and organisational units. Allocation of resources followed the same pathway. Despite successive management reforms in the late 1960s to early 1970s, this exposed key stressors in the organisation of health care. The difficulties in reconciling central funding and accountability, with the need to meet local needs were ever present (Ranade 1994). In addition, there was increasing medical autonomy over budgetary use; this reduced the effectiveness of central control. Government controlled the budget, but medicine continued to decide what to do with it.

After the 1979 general election, there was initially little alteration to the National Health Service (Klein 1983). However, poor economic growth, together with increasing public expenditure, gradually brought about changes. Influenced by the 'New Right' ideologies, a more interventionist, proactive, style of management in the health service emerged. This effectively changed the role of managers from one of reactive scapegoats for existing problems, to agents of the government (Flynn 1992). Managers became the means by which government control over NHS expenditure was increased (Harrison and Pollitt 1994).

The impetus for this change arose from the 1983 Griffiths report (NHS Executive 1983), a critique by the government health advisor, Sir Roy Griffiths. Within this report, four specific problem areas were identified: the limited management influence over the clinical professions; a managerial emphasis on reactivity to problems; the importance placed on managing the status quo; and a culture of producer, not consumer, orientation (Harrison et al. 1992).

The thrust of the Griffiths Report (*op. cit.*) was to challenge and restrict medicine's autonomy in the health service, and over health care resources. Indeed, nurses were only referred to twice throughout the document. Through its attention on organisational dynamics and not structure, the Griffiths Report proposed major change to the health service. General managers were introduced at all levels of the NHS. In spite of Griffiths' original intention that it was only cultural adjustment that was required, there were immediate and substantial structural and organisational changes in the health service (Robinson *et al.* 1989). Post-Griffiths there were increasing demands for value for money in the health service (DoH 1989). Attempts to extend managerial control over professional autonomy and behaviour therefore continued during this intense period of change, and culminated with the NHS and Community Care Act (DoH 1990).

From the re-organisations that occurred during this period, the NHS was restructured to conform more closely to the model of free enterprise in the private sector. This restructuring was shaped by the belief that greater efficiency could be engendered through the creation of an internal and competitive market. The belief that the health service was a distinctive organisation was disputed. The principles of economic rationality associated with business organisations were applied wholesale to the operation of health service. The services required were determined, negotiated, and agreed by purchasers and providers through a funding and contracting mechanism. In this, trust hospitals and Directly Managed Units supplied health care provision for District and General Practitioner fundholders.

There has since been a further shift in the purchaser base from health authorities to local commissioning through primary care groups (RCN 1998) and, more recently, through the *Shifting the Balance of Power: The Next Steps* policy document (DoH 2001b), to Primary Care Trusts. Through such established relationships, purchasers have become commissioners of services and the concept of the internal market has become the managed market that acknowledges the more long-term planning of services that is required. A rhetoric of partnership and health improvement underpins service agreements now made.

As this overview has demonstrated, the NHS is not only a technical institution for the delivery of care, but also a political institution where the practice of health care, and the roles of health care practitioners reflect the authority base within society. The hospital organisational structure is a powerful determinant of social identity, and thereby affects health care roles and responsibilities. However, through the health care reforms the medical staff and, to a lesser extent the managers, appeared to be buffered from the introduction of general management into the health service. This has resulted in health service delivery remaining strongly located within a medical model, and medical hegemony unchallenged (Mechanic 1991). It is the less powerful occupational groups, including nursing, that have felt the main impact of such reforms.

Working relationships: managers and health care professionals

The NHS organisational changes, as described in the preceding section, aimed to bring leadership, value for money, and professional accountability to managers at every level of the health service. These alterations were designed to reverse the organisational inertia that was restricting growth and efficiency in the system. Although originally intending a positive impact on the service, these revolutionary ideologies led to tension at the manager–health care professional interface (Owens and Glennerster 1990).

The introduction of the internal market in the NHS aimed to present a more neutral and efficient way of allocating resources, through rationalisation and depersonalisation. The new era of managerialism claimed to be a transforming force opposing traditional health professional power (Newman and Clarke 1994), and compelling professionals to submit to organisational objectives (Macara 1996). The conflicting models of health care held by managers and health care workers increased ambiguity over areas of responsibility and decision making, rather than clarity as intended (Owens and Glennerster 1990). The competing ideologies and tribalism between the health care groups were more explicitly revealed.

The introduction of markets to health care revealed a dichotomy for health care professionals. Medical and nursing staff were required to report to superior managerial officials, yet demonstrate professional allegiance to a collegial peer group. This was problematic, particularly for medical staff who understood medical authority and the autonomy of medical practice, but did not recognise managerial authority. In many of the commentaries addressing this, the most pragmatic solution to addressing this situation was to recognise that professional autonomy exists but together with, and limited, by administrative and managerial control (Elston 1991).

The medical management perspective

The Griffiths Report (NHS Management Executive 1983) considered the doctor as the natural manager and attempted to engage medicine with the general management ethos through the resource management initiative (Packwood et al. 1991). This required medicine to embrace the managerial values of collaboration, team work and collective achievement through the formation of clinical management teams: the clinical directorate. Conversely such working attitudes were in direct contrast to medicine's ideology of maximising rather than optimising, and of independence not interdependence (Moore 1990). It is interesting that even in today's health care environment, there have been continued observations that medical staff do not manage resources or clinical staff in a collegiate way (Audit Commission 1995, 1999). Despite this, there has been little attempt to undertake a systematic and comprehensive review of the organisation of medical work. This is in direct contrast to the experience of nurses, whose working practices and standards continue to be critiqued by all.

Early attempts made by managers to limit medical authority led to doctors adopting countervailing practices in order to remain autonomous and avoid organisational authority (Gable *et al.* 1994). Such practices, taken to protect their clinical autonomy, included discretionary behaviours in admitting patients or deciding on specific patient treatments (Harrison and Bruscini 1995, Freidson 1994). These behaviours rendered it difficult for managers to encroach on medical practice, and therefore limited the impact of the health care reforms.

Immediately post-Griffiths there was some evidence that introduction of general managers had, to a small extent, influenced medical practices. Green and Armstrong (1993) undertook a study on bed management in nine London hospitals. In this study, it was demonstrated how the work of administrative bed managers was able to influence throughput of patients, admission and operating lists, thereby indirectly affecting the work of medicine. Nonetheless, attempts made by managers to control medicine were self-limiting. Health care managers were not a monolithic, ideologically homogeneous group and lacked a strong cohesive power base (Harrison and Pollitt 1994). Managers did not fulfil their remit of challenging the medical position in the health service and avoided the responsibility for implementing unpleasant and difficult decisions (Harrison and Pollitt *op. cit.*).

The management ability of medicine continues to be challenged by government initiatives including the introduction of clinical governance (DoH 1997). In this, the Chief Executives of trusts are held accountable for the quality of clinical care delivered by the whole workforce. A positive impact of this change may be to provide opportunity for an integrated organisation with all team members, demonstrating an interdependent appreciation of health care (Marnoch and Ross 1998). Alternatively, it may be viewed as purely a structural change to increase the recognised authority of the Chief Executive over the traditional authority of medical staff: a further attempt to make in-roads into the medical power base.

Recent years have demonstrated continued commitment from the government towards modernising health care (DoH 2000b). This has included challenging traditional working patterns and clinical roles across clinical specialities and disciplines. Undoubtedly medicine has received increased public and government scrutiny over recent years. This has resulted in a shift of attitude from within and outside the medical profession. The success of challenging the agenda for change in health care will be part-determined by medicine's ability to further flex its own boundaries, and respond to the developing expertise of others. I suggest that the extent to which the current government health policy can be achieved, has yet to be determined.

The nursing–management perspective

The impact on nurses of the post-Griffiths health service structure has not been so insignificant. Empirical work has demonstrated that implementation of the Griffiths recommendations led to the removal of the nursing management structure. This effectively limited senior nurses to purely operational roles (Keen and Malby 1992). The implementation of the clinical directorate structure, with consultants having managerial accountability over nursing, further reduced nursing's ability to effect change (Levitt and Wall 1992).

Prior to 1984, budgetary control for nursing lay with the profession. The 1984 reorganisation 'removed nursing from nursing's own control and placed it firmly under the new general managers' (Robinson and Strong 1987, p. 5). As the concepts of cost containment and knowledgeable consumers were promoted, audit and accounting practices assumed an influential position in the health service. It was nurses who, comprising a significant percentage of the total workforce and associated staffing budget, found themselves targets for public and government scrutiny (Annandale 1996).

Nursing retained some strategic management functions within the new management structures, but these tasks were mainly restricted to areas within the professional nursing domain. Nurses have been seen as costly and potentially troublesome factors of production: channels through which costs can be decreased and administration functions can be absorbed (Ackroyd 1996). Caught in the crossfire of managerial changes that were initially targeted at medicine, nursing has been placed subordinate to management (Robinson and Strong 1987).

Despite debates on the impact of health care changes, there is consensus on one issue. The structural and organisational changes in the NHS since 1991 have re-fashioned unit management teams and unit management responsibilities. This has resulted in the increased involvement of these teams in the provision of the service. It has required a different way of thinking about health care, and new relationships between clinicians and managers to be developed (Owens and Glennerster 1990).

The clinical unit management team

One of the outcomes of the health service re-structuring was the creation of self-managing hospital trusts. The government centrally prescribed the composition of the executive boards that managed hospital trusts, but the organisational structure to manage the clinical units was left for local determination (Halford et al. 1997). The preferred model, developed in the 1990s, was the concept of the clinical directorate. This was based on the structure developed at the Johns Hopkins Hospital, United States of America.

The clinical directorate model was initially used in the UK at Guy's Hospital, London. This model was characterised by accountability, medical leadership, and executive control. In this way, the underpinning principles of the Griffiths Report were enacted at clinical unit level. The model sought to engage clinicians in the management process through a combined role of clinician-manager; the use of independent cost centres; and devolved budgets. Doctors almost exclusively led the clinical directorates as clinical directors. In these roles, medicine took responsibility for the unit management whilst retaining their clinical duties (Harwood and Boufford 1993). The clinical director was usually one role in a triadic structure. The other members of the unit management team generally included a business manager (career manager) and nurse manager (Fitzgerald 1994).

The principal clinical director role functions appeared to revolve around the co-ordination and development of clinical services; introducing quality standards and monitoring systems; implementing control of junior doctor hours; and managerial control over nurses and paramedics (Fitzgerald 1994). These managerial posts allowed medical staff to retain clinical autonomy and maintain professional allegiance to their collegiate peer group (Elston 1991). Many clinical directors took up these posts with little preparation or time commitment from trusts to undertake the required work for these posts. The nebulous role responsibilities, lack of remuneration and unclear selection processes caused initial reluctance amongst the medical staff to be appointed into these posts (Harwood and Boufford *op. cit.*).

There are studies now available to determine how medicine is functioning in these roles. A study by McKee *et al.* (1999) across six Scottish trusts provides a useful perspective with which to gauge the development of working relationships between medicine and managers. Using a postal questionnaire sent to clinical directors, together with follow-up interviews, this study demonstrated that the preferred style of medical management remained traditional and hierarchical. There were few real examples of managerial or power sharing models.

Mark and Dopson (1999) offers a slightly moderated position. Despite acknowledging that medicine and managers remain in polarised positions at trust level, examination of the clinical level reveals a more complex situation. Mark *et al.* (*op. cit.*) assert that there is evidence that new negotiations and alliances are being formed in the clinical areas. Concurring with Fitzgerald and Duffour (1997), it is suggested that this indicates a more collaborative form of working in the unit management team.

The nursing role in the management of the clinical unit has been poorly explored. Nursing input into unit management has only been highlighted specifically through the advanced and expert nurse literature. Through this, several important elements have been explored including organisational and work role competence (Benner 1984); consultation with physicians (Brykcznski 1989); collaboration and consultation (Hamric and Spross 1989); managerial authority (Thomson and Webster 1986); and policy making (Elliot 1995; O'Hanlon and Gibbon 1996).

Cohen's anthropological study (1995) undertaken during the introduction of the internal market system (1991–1993) is an exception to this. Data were collected through observation and interviews to examine the purchaser–provider split, contracting, and needs assessment in one English health authority. The contract negotiation process demonstrated variable involvement by medical staff, ranging from passive to proactive. Medical staff were seen to act in isolation from the team, acting as 'mavericks' (Cohen op. cit., p. 83). In this, examples were given of medical staff expressing their own personal views, and disrupting the agreed team and managerial strategies for contract negotiation.

Cohen (op. cit.) noted that nurses rarely spoke in contract negotiations, but were more involved in the drafting of the contract. In exploring the importance placed on developing a service policy with purchasers, nurses stressed the need to have clear articulation of nursing practice, with an emphasis on resources, professionalism, and quality in relation to patient need. Nurses were patient-oriented and had concerns for the involvement of user groups in relation to the description of the service. Given the clear interest nurses expressed in the process with the purchasers, the lack of nursing participation in the final negotiations was reflective of the marginality of nursing issues, and of nurses within the health service (Cohen 1995).

In acknowledging the emerging themes from this work, some caution must be exercised. The findings of this research must be read in the context in which it occurred, that is, within the first few years of the post-Griffiths structure. No interpretation or assumption can be made as to the roles and behaviours in contemporary unit management team: that requires further empirical work.

Since Cohen's study (op. cit.), further change has engulfed the NHS. Nurses in management positions are now charged to actively develop services with other lead clinicians through implementing national frameworks and engaging in debate and sharing with local clinical networks. These all require new working relationships to be developed with, amongst others, medical and managerial colleagues. Evaluation on the development and effectiveness of these relationships is not currently available. Additionally, there is little detail on performances by any member of the unit management team on the achievement of key competencies required of clinical managers.

The paucity of work on clinical unit management, and more specifically working relationships within this specific team is concerning. As previous chapters have demonstrated, there is great attention on team working at clinical patient level, but little on clinical management team working. This may be attributed to the lack of academic interest to examine this area, or lack of the necessary expertise to undertake the required research. Whilst this may be a potential explanation, it may more critically reflect the acceptance of medical and managerial dominance or the invisibility of nurses within unit management or the lack of empirical interest in nursing's contribution at this level.

The marginalised position that nurses have found themselves in the new management health care structures has been ascribed to the competing ideologies of the feminine values of nursing, with the masculine definition of the market and management styles (Davies 1996). It appears that as the gender relationship between the doctor and the nurse is becoming more egalitarian, this is being replaced by the gendered structures of new managerialism (Davies 1995). Nurses must choose to play the game or work to change the reference points.

Nursing and decision making at national policy level

It is recognised that gaining a better understanding of how nurses make decisions can impact on clinical and organisational effectiveness (Buckingham and Adams 2000). The decision-making literature has produced a wide range of clinical decision-making theories using diverse terminologies (Higgs and Jones 1995). The literature on clinical decision making focuses on several areas including probabilistic representation (Lilford et al. 1998) and pattern recognition judgements (Fonteyn 1999). This has resulted in distinctions being made on the processes that different health care professionals use to make clinical decisions (Crow et al. 1995). For example, use of the hypothetico-deductive approach, initially applied to medicine (Kassirer and Gorry 1978) has subsequently been applied to nursing (Taylor 1997).

However, such assertions need re-examination in today's environment when we are witnessing greater flexibility and development in health care roles. It is acknowledged that nursing work encompasses elements of medical, managerial and therapeutic work (Adams et al. 2000). From this, a common frame of reference for clinical decision making can contribute towards interdisciplinary collaboration, and engender greater understanding and accountability for decision making.

As these theories testify, decision making is a complex and potentially bewildering activity. It is too simplistic to think of clinical decision making as purely a series of cognitive, rational acts. As Thompson et al. (2000) highlight, there is little empirical work on the nature of decisions made by nurses in their everyday practice. This is particularly pertinent given the changing roles and the nature of interdisciplinary working. An exception of this is the work of Thompson et al. (2000) who used case study approach to understand the use of research in clinical decision making within acute medical and surgical ward areas. Decision making in the clinical context is acknowledged to be a social activity, often involving more than one clinician (Cioffi 2000). Therefore the social context in which the decision occurs also carries an impact. Clinical decision making is a dynamic activity involving interaction between individuals and the organisation within which they are located (Ham 1992).

For me, it is the organic, contextual factors influencing clinical decision making that are most interesting. The literature previously reviewed has debated the need for interdisciplinary communication in key decision-making forums, such as the ward round. Yet accounts of dominant medical behaviour and passive, under-confident nursing staff continue to proliferate. The political elements of clinical decision making are pivotal to understanding how medical and nursing staff work together to make clinical decisions. To begin to comprehend the micro-political influences at play, the literature on nursing participation in health policy offers some useful perspectives.

A specific definition of the term policy remains elusive, and its use remains ambiguous (Cheek and Gibson 1997). The Greek origin of the word 'polis' denotes citizenship or government (Oxford English Dictionary 1990). Policy refers to a process involved in taking decisions, producing statements, making plans, or developing an approach. Although there has been some confusion and academic debate regarding the differential use of the term policy and decision making, policy is generally associated with large-scale decisions made using a rational sequence (Hogwood and Gunn 1984). It therefore arises from a purposive concern, leading to a specific course of action (Anderson 1984). Health policy can therefore be defined as the 'managerial, collective or aggre-gated individual decisions which affect the way heath care is delivered . . . and includes care and treatment policies developed by professional and general managers' (Stacey 1991, p. 14).

The distinction between policy and decision making remain blurred, and the two are often used interchangeably. To date, two distinct positions have been taken in policy studies: the analysis of policy with its purpose to advance formal policy studies, and the analysis of policy with its more pragmatic focus (Ham and Hill 1986). I adopt the latter position throughout this text.

There have been different theoretical models put forward to explore policy. These have included: identification of the elements of the policy-making process, the levels of policy making in an organisation, and the effects of the policy process itself (Hogwood and Gunn 1984; Walt 1994). One of the most utilised of the functional models is Ham and Hill's policy process (1986). In this, the key areas of the policy process are formulation, implementation, and evaluation of the outcomes of policy. This linear model implies a degree of orderliness and consensus and that a way forward has been agreed and delineated.

Other theorists have analysed the policy process from a sociological perspec-tive taking into account the broader organisational, political, social relationships and influences (Barker 1996). For example, Alford (1975) used the concepts of pluralism, elitism, Marxism and structuralism to understand how power affects the policy process. Hall et al. (1975) developed this model further with an added category of bounded pluralism where major political, economic and health policy decisions are decided within a powerful elitist framework.

As inferred through these later works, policy is a political process occurring within an economic, interactional, value-laden context (Antrobus 1995). Although policy can be read as a linear process through some models, in reality, health policy is often created within a 'dynamic environment of competing forces and tensions' (Spurgeon 2000, p. 191) with policy actors receiving prominence over the policy processes itself (Walt 1994). This approach recognises that policy makers are not value free and, therefore, do not operate in a political vacuum.

Health care policy is a product of social and historical influences. Through this, policy represents the expressed values of the politically dominant group (Grimley 1986). It is therefore the vehicle that promotes the dominant group's ideology. Using this interpretation, any health care policy, from the development of National Service Frameworks to locally agreed patient treatment plans, can be read to understand the complex forces at work that compete to influence health care decisions at that level.

In sociological work, little attention had been paid to non-medical participants in health care. This has resulted in nursing policy studies being a relatively recent academic development (White 1988). Since the beginning of the 1960s, scrutinisation of the work of non-medical occupations has gradually increased. This is at the level of individual occupations, and in relation to medicine. The effect of feminism, and an increased awareness of the high level of complexity in health care labour have been key influential factors in this (Elston 1991).

More recently, the analysis of nursing has shifted from its location in a discrete academic field, to the analysis of nursing in the overall division of labour, and in the negotiation of occupational boundaries on care. This re-conceptualisation of the health care occupations has heralded a change in the perception of medical power and challenged nursing's position as a suppressed occupational subspecies (Salvage 1988). Policy issues in nursing have therefore provided avenues to explore and clarify power issues associated with the delivery of a nursing service within the health care system (Robinson 1997).

Despite this increased awareness, nursing remains marginalised within the health care policy process. Policy studies continue to render nursing invisible, focusing predominantly on the medical and managerial contribution (Walby and Greenwall 1994). There continues to be an unequal representation of nursing and medicine within the policy development. At all levels of the policy-making process, medical staff are the major resource consumers, providers and controllers of health care (Ham 1992). Medical staff involvement in health care policy is, therefore, well established through representation at government (Masterson 1994) through to clinical unit level (Antrobus 1995).

In policy terms, nurses continue to operate in a 'black hole' (Robinson 1997, p. 251). Nurses remain unable to see their work within a broader policy context, and therefore have negligible contribution to the policy process. Equally, there continues to be little insight and response by medical and managerial colleagues to nursing developments or concerns. It is only through transformation of nursing issues into a crisis that nursing problems receive attention and reach the policy agenda (Robinson et al. 1993). The national recruitment problems in nursing (Audit Commission 1999) and development of nursing practices in response to medical staff shortages are clear examples of this.

To date, there has been little contemporary, empirical, work undertaken on the role of the nurse in decision making at any level. Much of the policy work is to be found in discussion papers. In the majority of policy studies undertaken at clinical unit level, medicine and managers appear to be the only players. This renders critical analysis and synthesis of the nursing involvement in clinical management policy difficult, without merely adding to the pool of rhetoric and opinion. Despite such an empirical omission, there is still resounding governmental support for nurses to be involved in the policy process and to contribute to service delivery decisions (DoH 1999, 2000b). This must therefore make this area an important consideration for study.

Nurses, midwives and health visitors comprise the biggest staff group of health professionals employed by the NHS (DoH 1999). It is therefore understandable that the nature of nursing work and the nursing group are often on the receiving end of health care policy developments (Masterson 2002). Given the continued impetus from the government towards democratic health care teams, flexible role boundaries and new ways of working, other issues are less explicable. In exploring the contribution of all practitioners across health care, the maintained profile of medicine with lack of input from other health care workers remains indefensible. It is to explore this situation and stimulate debate that this book is directed.

Chapter 4

The study

This chapter describes the study on which this book is based. The purpose of this chapter is not to detail and critique the research approach used. Instead, I have selectively explored elements of the study to enable the rigour of the work to be judged. Therefore, I will outline the research method and sampling approach, and then describe the data collection methods that I used in the field.

A second, and important function of this chapter is to give the reader insight into the challenges that I experienced when researching in the social world of clinical practice. Through this, I hope that both social scientists and health care practitioners can share and understand some of my experiences. To this end, I do not engage in academic debate about the data analysis model adopted. Instead, I spend a substantial amount of time exploring the complexity of data collection in the field, and on the nature of fieldwork ethics in a clinical setting.

From the outset of the study, it was clear to me that to appreciate clinical decision making, I had to understand how nurses and doctors work in a clinical area. To achieve this, I chose an ethnographic research approach as defined by Atkinson and Hammersley. In this, ethnography is:

> a strong emphasis on exploring the particular phenomena, rather than setting out to test hypotheses about them; a tendency to work primarily with 'unstructured data', that is, data that have not been coded at the point of data collection in terms of a closed set of analytic categories; investigation of a small number of cases . . .; analysis of data that involves explicit interpretation of the meanings and functions of human actions, the product of which mainly takes the form of verbal descriptions, with quantification and statistical analysis playing a subordinate role at most.
>
> (Atkinson and Hammersley 1994, p. 248)

In ethnography, in order to explore the phenomena and the alternate realities that exist, thick description of the culture occurs through data that are collected in the field and described in depth, and over time (Geertz 1973). In order to achieve this, I used three specific data sources of cultural information: cultural behaviour from what people do; cultural artefacts from what people make or use; and speech messages from what people say (Spradley 1980). The main methods that I used to collect such data were, therefore, participant observation, cultural documents and ethnographic interviews (Wolcott 1994).

The study I present here is a descriptive ethnography. In this, I used three intensive care sites located within England. My initial case selection was purposeful (Sandelowski *et al.* 1992) and I chose sample sites in anticipation of their ability to provide rich information about the research focus. After I had gained ethical approval and access, I collected data during 1998–2000.

I adopted a reflexive approach in this study. Through this, I recognised that, in undertaking the research, I was part of the social world under study. In the following sections I will therefore make my role in the research process explicit so that 'rather than engaging in futile attempts to eliminate the effects of the researcher we should set about understanding them' (Hammersley and Atkinson 1983, p. 17). Throughout this book, I make my intentions transparent with explicit reference to, and ownership of, personal thoughts and influences. These are then open to the reader as part of the analysis.

Gaining access to the field

Whilst gaining access to the field is a critical component of the research process, it has only received attention in relatively recent times (Moser and Kalton 1983). As noted by Burgess (1984), access can be a complex procedure requiring negotiation and renegotiation. It often marks a rite of passage for any ethnographic work.

In this work, I chose the senior nurse as the first point of contact in approaching the intensive care units. Without the support of this key gatekeeper, I perceived that access would not be granted. I saw the senior nurse as a potential valuable 'sponsor' and supporter of my research; one who would be an ally in the system. Initial contact with the senior nurse was made by telephone, which I then followed with a more formal meeting. The agenda for this meeting was to discuss the study, the nature of the data collection, and the research outcomes for the unit. Following these meetings, I sent a letter detailing the outline of the research to the senior nurse and others in the clinical team who had expressed an interest. Once initial contact had been established, I found that each field site was unique in the procedure that I used to gain access and ethical approval. As Adler and Adler (1987) observed, gaining access was situationally specific.

Gaining physical access to a research site is an acknowledged precondition for social access to field sites. However, social access, gaining consent to observe individuals in the field, brings other challenges to address (Dingwall 1980). Although the senior staff, as gatekeepers, had given their consent for the research, my participant observation fieldwork required me to work alongside more junior staff. In this, I needed to give consideration as to how I could impart more general information about the study prior to field entry, and the more detailed information required to negotiate day-to-day access on the units.

Therefore, I used study outlines, presented at staff meetings, met with managers, and left information about the study in unit communication books, prior to field entry. Once in the field, I used particular progressive entry strategies (Johnson 1975) in order to identify forums and staff to link with. On a day-to-day basis, I began discussions with the nurse in charge to identify participant observation opportunities for the next day. Such opportunities included attendance on the ward round, working alongside staff and attending unit management meetings.

It was crucially important that I gave consideration to staff, patient and families in the sites. I had no involvement with any particularly intrusive situations, for example in caring for the dying patient and their family. This was consistent with personal and professional philosophy of respect for, and sensitivity to, individual needs. Once a staff member had been identified for the next day, I then approached them and explained my research, the purpose of my observations together with an explicit statement about my role. I always presented an 'opt out' clause ('You may have had others working with you recently – so you may want a break – that's OK'). This proved a pragmatic and opportunistic sampling strategy (Burgess 1984) to negotiate daily access. I then returned to that person before the end of the shift for their decision.

In the literature on gaining social access, issues of overt or covert research, and conditional access are often debated (Burgess 1984; Hammersley and Atkinson 1995). My own personal values did not favour a covert research approach, and I felt that my professional background enabled my presentation to be open and honest. I particularly found expressing a want to 'uncover their side of the story' a useful phrase. I worked hard at developing a rapport with all staff, demonstrating an understanding of the environment, and of not abusing my position. As a result, there were few restrictions placed on this research or my role as researcher.

One issue that naively I did not consider, were any field site agendas. As discussed by Lee (1993), the motives of gatekeepers in engaging in research are not often explored. In this study, I did not feel that any such issues were initially apparent. Nevertheless, on returning to the research sites to discuss the initial findings and dissemination strategies, I found overwhelming expectations of my research that needed careful management. This is revealed in the following fieldwork journal excerpt:

> I feel as if they want me to provide them with all the answers . . . there are unrealistic expectations that I am going to provide them with solutions to all their problems . . . I have to re-iterate the aims and the purpose of the research over again, I have to be very clear in what I can and cannot deliver.

Data collection methods

Ethnography is both a process and a product of research (Agar 1980). In this, there are three fundamental characteristics: the researcher as an instrument observing, collecting and recording cultural data, the fieldwork, and the cyclical nature of data collection and analysis (Hammersley and Atkinson 1995). As noted earlier, I used participant observation, interviewing and use of documentary sources as key data collection methods in this study.

Through participant observation, I was able to participate in the 'daily life of the group . . . enter into conversation with some or all . . . and discover their interpretations of the events' (Becker 1958, p. 652). I predominantly adopted the role of observer as participant (Gold 1958) for this study, although I needed to be flexible in this role. My rationale for adopting this approach was to ensure that I minimised the risk of going native in the clinical areas. In this way, my research and the research questions I had remained central to my observations, and I did not become distracted by the clinical situations and details.

In all the sites, a pattern of engagement occurred. In order to enculture myself into that unit, my initial role could be described as complete participant. Once established on the unit, I adopted a role more consistent with that of 'observer as participant' and then towards the end of the fieldwork, more of an observer role, to indicate a closure and withdrawal from that site. This pattern for the initial stage, phase 1 of the study, is demonstrated in Figure 4.1.

In the ethnographic interviews, I was mindful of Burgess's (1984) description of qualitative interviews as conversations with purpose, showing many features of a friendly conversation (Spradley 1980). A semi-structured interview guide, generated by the original research questions, was used. This had flexibility to allow exploration of issues raised by the participants, or from other aspects of the fieldwork (Barriball and While 1994). The interviews that occurred in this study were formal, taped interviews and the more opportunistic informal interviews that occurred spontaneously on the clinical units.

I used Spradley's (1979) framework of ethnographic questions to structure the interviews. This logical, progressively analytical approach to question construction is similar to Krueger's funnelling procedure (1994). Three types of ethnographic questions were used. The interview opened with a non-threatening, grand tour, descriptive question. This was followed by a more specific, structural question to explore basic domains of cultural knowledge. Contrast questions were then used to discover, through presentation of conflicting situations, cultural meaning for the participant. This was achieved by emphasising similarities and differences in how participants saw their world. As highlighted in the literature (Chenitz and Swanson 1986, Holloway and Wheeler 1996), the general principles of interviewing were familiar to me through my work as a nurse. I found the use of echo, reflective and affirmative probes particularly useful to explore areas exposed by study participants.

Chenitz and Swanson (1986) also identify informal interviews as being a useful and effective source of data. In this research, informal interviews were

Participant role

Fieldwork stage	Duration	Purpose	Fieldwork strategies
I	1 week	• personal introductions • orientation to unit • fieldwork planning	• aim for high unit profile • work clinical shifts • work with staff in assisting in care • wear 'uniform' • identify key participants and forums • book key appointments • identify key documentary sources
II	2 weeks	• key data collection: – participant observation – ethnographic interviews	• maintain unit profile • work predominantly clinical shifts • attend key policy forums • wear 'uniform' • interview key participants
III	1 week	• documentary data collection • closure and withdrawal from unit	• remaining ethnographic interviews • collection of documentary data • work office hours • wear non-clinical clothes • appointment to thank key participants and staff • agree return dates • follow-up letter of thanks

Observer role

Figure 4.1 Fieldwork, phase 1

the brief, natural conversations that occurred during participant observation. I found that these interviews required a more conscious use of myself and of my interpersonal skills, in order to engage others in conversation. It required a sensitivity to cultural norms and rules to know when, where and how to approach potential participants. Due to the unstructured nature of the informal field interviews, I chronicled these as brief, key sentences or words in my fieldwork journal so that I could capture the essence of the interview. I then expanded on these notes at the earliest opportunity.

Despite the importance of documents in informing practical and political decisions (May 1993), little use has been made of this data source (Plummer 1990). In the study, I viewed documents as social products: artefacts produced by the organisation or group. As such I was able to examine them critically in order to identify representations of an independent reality (Hammersley and Atkinson 1995). A range of organisational documents was used in this way, including literature in the public domain (patient information leaflets and trust reports); formal organisational literature (trust business plan, policies and organisational plans); and formal unit literature (nursing care plans, job descriptions, and minutes from meetings).

Over the three sites, a total of eighteen taped ethnographic interviews was obtained, more than seven hundred and twenty hours of participant observation took place, including informal interviews, and sixty-two documents were collected and used in the data analysis.

The fieldwork role

As discussed earlier, the predominant researcher role adopted in this study could broadly be described as observer as participant. I found that this was most applicable to ensure that I could best manage the marginal position between the two worlds of the researched and the researcher (Hammersley and Atkinson 1995). In acknowledging that the social researcher actively participates in the social situation (Hammersley and Atkinson 1995), I needed to be reflexive throughout my field experiences. This section details issues concerning role management and identification in the field.

As mentioned previously, there were few limitations placed on my field role, although I did not attend some of the management meetings in one site as some had only recently been established and were of a sensitive nature. In the field, my main responsibilities were assisting the unit team in procedures and helping with basic patient care and general housekeeping during busy times (Reid 1991). It was providing such general assistance that heightened my unit profile, and helped me to identify potential study opportunities. Half way through the data collection period, I asked for feedback from senior nurses on my role. I worked hard at my fieldwork role, and at my character display (van Maanen *et al.* 1982) and subsequently my role was well received in all sites.

The fieldwork was managed so that I initially worked alongside the nursing staff, and later the medical staff. I ensured that I was at all nursing handovers so that I could introduce myself to the nursing team and develop a rapport with all staff. During the handover time, I met up with the key link person on the unit for that day. As most of the beds were arranged in three and four bed bays, not only was the link nurse a participant in the study, but I could also assist other staff and, therefore, engage them in conversation about the research area. I found this to be a useful strategy giving flexibility to both researcher and participants. Where I decided to place myself on the unit for the day was also a consideration. Once I became familiar with the unit and key data collection opportunities, I realised that a conscious positioning of myself was important. On all units, for example, the ward round inevitably started from one place, either a specific bed or from the nurses' station. I therefore chose to work in an area that had a direct view out to this vantage point.

As highlighted in the literature (Smart 1984; Gerrish 1997), my dress and appearance was a prior consideration for the fieldwork. As I planned to work with nurses and undertake some basic care, I needed a uniform to allow me to assist safely in care. I also needed to be distinguishable from the permanent staff. After discussions with the site senior nurses, I wore theatre blues when undertaking clinical work. Towards the end of the field period when concentrating on obtaining final interviews and documentation, I wore smart casual wear as I felt this sent messages of closure in that site. It was also important that I could be clearly recognised. Ensuring clear identification was important, both as a courtesy to others and in limiting deception.

In each site, I worked four days a week in the field: three clinical shifts and one day writing up expanded field notes and undertaking administrative work for the next week's field visit. I worked a mixture of shifts that covered a twenty-four hour period. Within each shift, I developed a daily schedule that allowed for periods of writing up field notes. This was undertaken away from the 'public' unit, and occurred in unit offices or staff rooms when these were not in use. I found that short periods of observation followed by writing up were most conducive to remaining alert and producing detailed field accounts. In addition, in undertaking fieldwork in my own culture, there was a particular need to focus on the mundane, and not the exotic or atypical (Berg 1989). Use of Spradley's (1980) framework and developing geographical site and decision-making forum maps were also useful to maintain rigorous descriptive detail.

The field record

To ensure that all observations could be recorded in an accessible, logical and thorough manner, I recorded all data in a fieldwork journal (Burgess 1984). Substantive, methodological and analytical field notes were made located in a single journal. The substantive field notes were the descriptive record of observed situations, events and conversations in the field (Bogdan and Biklen 1982). These were combined with ethnographic interviews and documentation to form the primary data sources. Some ethnographers have developed structured forms for substantive notes (Humphrey 1970). I found that using a 'free text' approach was a more natural approach to description in the field.

My methodological notes encompassed the reflective components on the researcher role, field experiences and the research method. This approach, promoted by Malinowski (1922) and Geer (1964), became the basis of the reflexive elements I used throughout this study. The analytical notes written in the field represented my preliminary thoughts on data analysis. As grounded theory underpinned the data analytical process, these analytical notes were seen as contributing to the more formal component of analytic memos (Glaser and Strauss 1967). I found that writing a summary of key events, repeated themes and concepts at the end of each day a useful exercise to adopt.

In reality, the fieldwork notes took several forms. Whilst actually in the field, I made use of a small pocket notebook and a dictaphone in which I could note key phrases or words. During the periods in my daily schedule for making field notes, I developed these into larger expanded accounts. Whilst Burgess (1984) has recommended that the three types of field notes data are kept separate, I preferred to keep them all located together in a large fieldwork journal, but with a clear indexing system. I saw this as a 'living document' of the field, in which my observations, reflections and embryonic analytic thoughts were all recorded, as they occurred chronologically and in context.

Data analysis model

Ethnographic data analysis has been identified as being vague, intuitive and researcher driven (LeCompte and Goetz 1982). I therefore developed a three stage model of data analysis (Figure 4.2) in order to provide structure and rigour to this process. This model of data analysis utilised the constant comparative method (Glaser and Strauss 1967), and upheld the general analytical principles espoused by Hammersley and Atkinson (1983). To achieve density and rigour in the work, I used analytical memos with definitions and descriptions of the major properties of the developing categories. Miles and Huberman's work (1994) informed data presentation through diagrams that I used to illustrate developing concepts and to provide a useful tool to reflect on the theoretical evolution of the study. A computer package (Ethnograph 4.0) was used to aid data coding and data management. Whilst this particular system had some recognised limitations, I had a local support network of other ethnographers who all had familiarity and expertise with this software.

Protection of participants

Ethical consent is particularly difficult in naturalistic research where informed consent from all participants is complex and potentially problematic (Merrell and Williams 1994). However, throughout this research I made every attempt to avoid and limit deception. This required me to be honest and truthful at all stages. This has been explored previously in negotiating access and managing the researcher role.

In order to protect the autonomy of the participants, it was important that I gave information about the research, so that informed consent could be achieved. I used such strategies as written and verbal information giving; allowing time for questioning; time for consideration of the research (by the unit, key gatekeepers and individual staff); and letting people know that 'no' to my requests was their right. As I have discussed earlier in this chapter, there was also a need for me to be sensitive to the wider political and personal issues in the field. It was equally important for me to iterate that the study was not intended to be judgemental about the quality of input into clinical decision making or about the quality of care *per se*, but was to understand how clinical decisions were made on that unit.

Social research, in attempting to understand cultural life, has the potential to be intrusive. Limiting imposition was, therefore, important. My management of the researcher role, my interpersonal skills and an awareness of the culture under study enabled me to be informed and responsive. The development of trust and respect with key gatekeepers allowed information to be obtained through the most suitable and least invasive means of data collection. In agreeing with Lathlean (1996b), I chose not to use the unguarded, unofficial but potentially data-rich, coffee room conversations. I preferred to raise such issues during

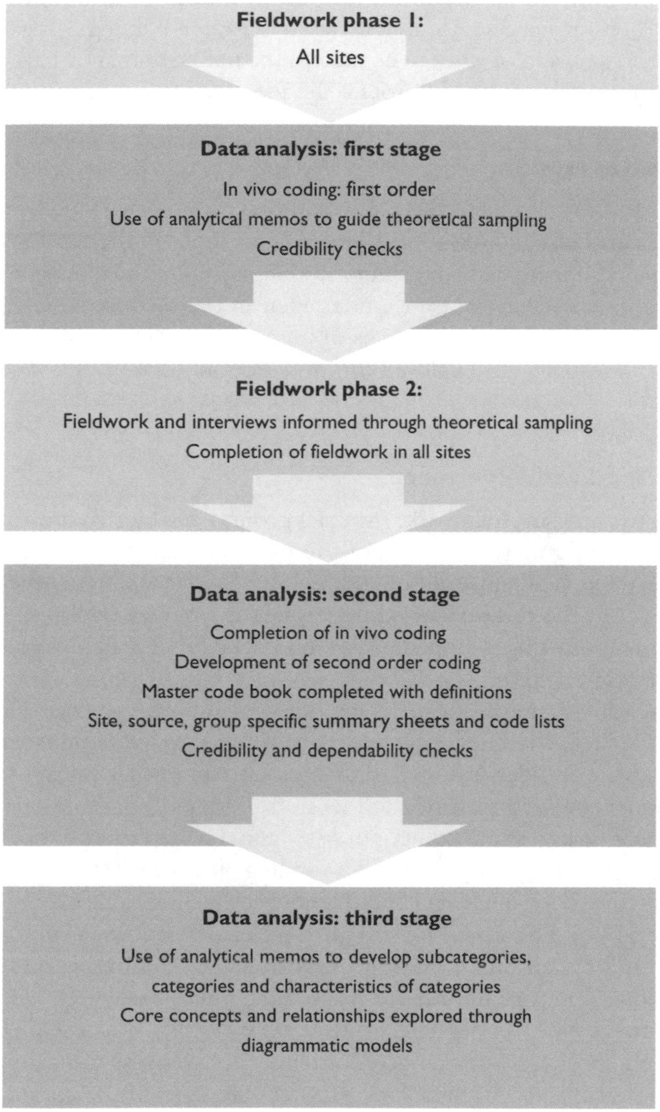

Figure 4.2 Data analysis model

the subsequent periods of field observation, and allow participants to knowingly consent to discussion of such areas.

Issues of confidentiality and anonymity in the use of the findings were more problematic. Whilst I could uphold confidentiality, trying to maintain anonymity was more problematic with the choice of an ICU nursing development unit as a sample site. As such units are few in number, this site could be identified.

When I raised this explicit concern with the unit, it transpired to not being an issue for them. After further discussions with all sites, I agreed strategies regarding the inclusion and exclusion of work to be used in the public domain. I have tried to remain true to the data texts, but protect the identity of participants.

Personal reflections

The final section of this chapter offers a personal narrative on two specific issues that became of particular interest to me. This section looks at the tensions that two particular situations created. An exploration of managing the researcher role whilst being an intensive care nurse is undertaken in the section 'Researching the lived experience', and my perceptions of managing my clinical role whilst being a social researcher is explored in the section 'Living the research experience'.

Researching the lived experience

On preparing to start my fieldwork, my background reading cautioned me against the hazards of going native, and of the need to manage marginality in the role of researcher (Lofland and Lofland 1995). I therefore entered the field attempting to adopt the position of ethnographer as stranger (Delamont and Atkinson 1995). From this, I hoped that I could begin my fieldwork with cultural naiveté (Geer 1964).

During this study, I was a social researcher researching my own clinical speciality. Yet, it felt as if I was being constantly challenged to live simultaneously in two worlds: as an outsider (researcher) and yet also an insider (nurse) to the social world under study. To manage such tensions I adopted the role of a new member of the nursing team, someone with general experience but who required clarification of any 'jargon' used. This strategy has been detailed in other works and worked well for me, even if it did render me feeling somewhat 'stupid' (Reid 1991, p. 547). I also aimed for a high level of descriptive accuracy and artificial naiveté (Stephenson and Greer 1981) in all my field notes and used Spradley's (1980) framework in order to make the familiar strange.

There were times when I concurred with Coffey (1999), in that stating that I could adopt the position of estranged ethnographer was just too simplistic, and ignored the complexity of fieldwork. Having taken great time considering and negotiating the field role, there continued to be incidents for which I had not planned. These directly revealed tensions between my role as professional nurse and as social researcher. In one incident, I was working alongside a nurse caring for a lady. I had introduced myself to the patient's daughter and she knew that I did not work on the unit but was undertaking research. I wrote in my fieldwork notes:

> The nurse looking after the patient next door then came over and berated the daughter for not having her shoes on due to the infection risk from the

floor. The daughter explained she had recently had a foot operation and needed to walk barefoot if possible to exercise her feet. The conversation terminated and the nurse then went next door to give care. The daughter sat down and I noticed she was tearful. I got her some tissues and sat with her, and she started to talk: the pressure of her mother's illness and being 'the doctor' in the family [she was a GP] was too much. She asked me questions about her mother's progress and I said she needed to ask the unit nurse and I suggested she would be back soon. She thanked me but then said 'I think you ought to speak to your colleague about her attitude' . . . I was speechless, I could understand what had driven her to say that and why at this time. But as this was my first day at this field site, my mind was racing from wanting to empower this relative, to support her at this distressing time, and yet stay in the researcher role.

My distress and feeling incompetent at managing this incident is documented. I was acutely aware of the dimensions of the situation, and the roles impacting on my interpretation of this incident. Some consolation came from the auto-biographical account in Whyte's *Street Corner Society* (1981), from which I realised that my naiveté with regards to managing fieldwork was shared. When reflecting on this event, I determined that throughout the fieldwork if the situation required, I would offer minimal, but sympathetic intervention. I would also respond to human need, not as a member of the nursing team, but as a fellow human being. This included listening and being supportive, but not making judgements or passing comment. Each time I found myself in such complex situations, I was continually reminded of Williams's (1990b) comment that researcher role boundaries are never as clear as in research reports.

The second incident occurred when I realised before other staff, that one patient was going into cardiac arrest:

> I was helping a nurse look after a lady who was very sick and I noted that no plan or treatment had been made on the ward round regarding withdrawal of treatment. From my professional perspective, it was fairly clear that this lady was going to arrest. As I was talking to the nurse, I became aware that there were [pre-terminal] cardiac rhythm disturbances. I was concerned that this lady was going to suffer, in my opinion, the further indignity of a full resuscitation.

I then continued to document my deliberate and progressive actions on attempting to indicate my concerns to the nurse. These were particularly prompted as the lady's son had just gone to the canteen for lunch. The nurse did not share my concerns and I was informed: 'Oh, don't worry, she'll go on for ages yet.' My fieldwork journal continues:

> I reflected on this afterwards, worrying that I had overstepped the boundaries of researcher role. My actions were prompted by the strong desire for

respect for the lady and my professional ethics. The situation was literally life threatening and I felt compelled to do something. After talking to the staff involved, I do not feel that any of the staff felt threatened by my actions, and that the patient herself had not unduly suffered by my interventions.

In working through these particular situations, I established several further fieldwork guidelines to add to those previously negotiated with the senior nurses. I felt that whilst I was not a practising nurse on that unit, I was a practising nurse on the professional register and therefore, honour my professional duty to care. My professional duty would be exercised sensitively, as the situation required. This required me to intervene professionally and assist if others were not in a position to intervene, but to withdraw as soon as safely possible.

The final strategy, concurring with Davis (1992), was that if intervention did occur, there needed to be awareness that it had occurred, why it occurred, and the effect that this had. In taking this stance, it became clear that the researcher role in the field was complex and multi-faceted. In negotiating such field incidents, rather than become the ethnographer as stranger on the periphery of the field, I became located in the midst in the field. Through this, fieldwork became conceptualised as an active and (inter)personal process. In finding resolution to such challenges, it became apparent that it was important to remain reflexive about my fieldwork experiences. I had to realise what expectations and experiences I brought with me, and others' expectations of me. One incident revealed this well. After having coffee with two of the consultants on one site and feeling that the meeting had gone well, we walked back to the unit. The following comment was then made: 'So OK, do we have to do anything special whilst you're here then?'

I found that, similar to Atkinson (1997), the need to manage relations with those in the field required the use of my health care knowledge. My relationship with those in the field was managed and recast, dependent on the participant I was working with. On working with a junior member of staff, I consciously iterated the need to explain to me how things were done here. This not only ensured accuracy in my field notes but also was an attempt to minimise any perceived power differential. With consultants and senior nurses, the interviews were more relaxed and similar to having a conversation with a peer.

It was not only perceptions about my professional role that were challenged during the fieldwork. I found my role as woman and as human being challenged. For me, one experience became an 'epiphany moment' (Denzin 1992), one which truly revealed the complexity of reflexivity. In one site, I had arranged to meet a consultant in what I assumed to be his offices, located near theatres. He gave me directions and following these I was led into theatres, not his office, but directly into a gynaecological theatre list. As I later wrote in my fieldwork journal:

I just couldn't believe it, I was not prepared for it. So many things going through my head. Most importantly, feeling for the woman on the operating table, in surely the most undignified of all positions – and another stranger – me – in the room. Concern that if we were to talk in the theatre, would he concentrate on his list? Would others be able to hear our conversation? I just couldn't believe it.

In recounting this, I knew that I was bringing all sorts of judgements and experiences to bear on this event: my own experiences as a woman, a nurse, a researcher, and as a human being. It was only that by identifying these influences that I could make sense of the emotions experienced, identify the lessons learnt, and then make explicit the influences on the data collected. The insight derived from this incident made me conscious of the different roles adopted as a researcher in the field, and in the field notes (Rudge 1996). It made me more cognisant of how I located myself in the study (Stanley and Wise 1983), and the assertions made about being a practising nurse. It made me become critical as to why those assertions were made, and of my own need to create and construct a personal and political piece of writing.

Managing the researcher role in fieldwork was undoubtedly stressful. It required total commitment and energy to the research, and to maintaining critical awareness of one's role. The personal involvement and responsibility to the fieldwork led, at the end of a week in the field, to feeling physically and emotionally tired. There were some incidents in the field that left me distressed and shocked. Such events made me question not only the ethics of medicine, but those of my nursing colleagues. I could readily identify with the emotional nature of fieldwork as reflected in Cannon's (1989) account of her work with breast cancer patients, and Burr's (1996) in-depth interviews with spouses of intensive care families.

There were considerable challenges in managing the field role, but I was extremely fortunate in all the units who agreed to take part in my study. During the entire fieldwork period, staff were always giving of their time, and always willing to talk to me. Experiences gained in the field acted as my *rite of passage* into ethnographic fieldwork. I made new acquaintances, gained new insights, and have been privileged in some small way, to care for and about people. It is experiences such as these, which made researching the lived experience such a rewarding and enlightening encounter.

Living the research experience

Hammersley and Atkinson (1995) have commented that one rarely leaves the field unaffected, and this remains poorly documented (Wolcott 1990). Whilst undertaking this research, I continued to practise one day a week in my home unit. In this, I continued to care for patients and, on a shift to shift basis, manage the unit as required. I therefore considered whether undertaking research in clinical decision making, an area I constantly confronted during my clinical shifts, had influenced my nursing role. I also considered how my experiences of using an ethnographic approach had affected my view about the health care environment within which I worked. In this section I explore the issue of how living the research experience, has changed me as a clinical nurse in intensive care.

I have always been clear about the circumstances that led me to study the area of clinical decision making in intensive care. For me, the research problems arose from practice as explored in the introductory chapter. I was looking for understanding and solutions that could be used to address such practice issues. What perhaps, was not made so clear, were the 'ghosts of other ethnographies' (Williams 1990b, p. 3).

Two years on from the research, I can now see the influence of my academic curiosity reflected in the professional and sociological interest areas of these early chapters. My final choice of the study area and research approach was influenced by my personal philosophies. For example, neither Marxist nor feminist thought has a distinct profile in this study. I can track how, during the planning phase of this work, my focus developed from an advanced practice perspective, to an ethics perspective on accountability, and finally on decision making. I became increasingly aware of how I located my experiences and myself throughout the study. The research process was rigorous and analytical, but I can see the influence of personal and professional practice on the orientation of this study.

The question was if, or how this study and the resultant field experiences would influence my practice? It was no surprise to me, that in using an ethnographic approach I became more aware of understanding others' points of view, of acknowledging that there were multiple realities. I considered the context of the situation more, of seeing the viewpoint of all those involved, before acting. I integrated sociological concepts into my worldview. Initially, it made me almost become impotent in my thinking, and wondering what really was the 'right' way to proceed. As in this fieldwork entry, I appeared to be experiencing Porter's 'praxial paralysis' (Porter 1996, p. 76):

> How does one move on? If there are multiple realities here – how does this help me in managing this situation? A doctor wants to admit a 76-year-old woman with severe chronic respiratory disease and pneumonia, because he feels the chest infection is treatable and that this episode can be cured. But the nursing staff, including myself, does not agree. I think the poor woman will be with us for days on end and never get off the ventilator – how has my understanding of these realities helped this woman?

During this time, it also became obvious to me that the values underpinning collaborative working practices were not just evident in my clinical practice. I became aware of my preferred style of addressing academic, professional and personal debate. I believe that undertaking the research, has indeed created 'ripples on the self' (Ely et al. 1997, p. 329) and led to personal change and development.

All researchers have a desire to make comments on those we study; this is surely the focus of any research. What is equally important to acknowledge, is that in doing so, we say something about ourselves. In this way, 'our research tells a story about ourselves' (Steier 1995, p. 3).

Chapter 5

Understanding the context

This chapter sits between presentation of the study and the main chapters that explore key issues relating to clinical decision making in intensive care. In this chapter I set the scene so that the reader can understand the context within which decision making occurred. There are two elements to this. The first is to have a familiarity with the settings within which this work was undertaken. To this end, in the first half of the chapter I describe the specific clinical units. In this, I will describe the units with details about their size, clinical services offered together with any general observations made while I was undertaking fieldwork. Any specific projects or developments that occurred on the unit during the study and that I used to explore interdisciplinary working are also made explicit.

In the second half of this chapter I explore the clinical and service management forums within which decisions were made. The types of forums, and their structure and membership are reviewed. I hope that in taking some time to explore such essential background detail, the stage will be set to address the key matters arising from this work.

The clinical sites

As outlined in the previous chapter, all three of the clinical units used in this study were classified as general intensive care units. One site was a large university teaching hospital unit with complex service configurations and regional services and one was a district general hospital site. This mix, despite offering broadly similar clinical services, demonstrated variation in terms of the size of the unit and clinical speciality services offered. The third site was chosen as it was an established nursing development unit (NDU). These clinical units, with a nursing centred philosophy, have a strong focus on clinical nursing, education, and research developments within a facilitative, non-hierarchical structure (Manley 1990; Mills 1997). The inclusion of an intensive care nursing development unit, therefore, gave opportunities to explore whether developing a prominent nursing culture altered in any way the dynamics of how doctors and nurses work to make decisions. This site acted as a case for analysis, demonstrating variance from the other two. Each of these sites is now described in some depth.

Site 1

This site was located in an older established building. In the hospital literature made available for the public, the trust described itself as 'one of the premier clinical, teaching and research centres in the country with an international standing'. The intensive care unit was located within the surgical division, one of the four clinical divisions within the trust. In the surgical division there were nine other clinical services including cardiac, trauma, dental, private patients and theatres. The service management of the ICU was led by a clinical director of ICU (consultant), a unit manager (nurse manager), and a clinical nurse specialist (lead nurse).

The ICU was found in a previous ward area, located near to theatres and the cardiac services areas. The doors of the unit were secured, so staff gained entry through knowing the combination lock number, and visitors used an intercom system to talk to staff who then opened the front doors of the unit. As with all older hospital buildings, space was at a premium and ward areas had been refurbished to enable services to be delivered. The unit was actually spread out over a large geographical area. This comprised a mixture of single cubicles, four and six bedded bays and separate rooms. Indeed, this geographical layout caused problems for both nursing and medical staff in observing patients, managing the unit, and in supporting staff to deliver care. It was clear that all had recognised the problems caused by the lack of space and there were plans for further hospital redevelopment onto a new development site.

The main clinical unit on this site had eighteen intensive care beds. The beds were designated as six high dependency beds, four beds for patients requiring overnight ventilation, and eight intensive care beds. The beds for overnight ventilation were primarily intended for patients who had undergone cardiac surgery. The majority of such patients required short-term ventilation before returning to the cardiac ward areas the next day. Similar to the other sites, the unit also cared for patients requiring admission after general surgery and for emergency treatment of medical disorders. Although no children were cared for on this unit, and the emergency department was located on a satellite site, I counted a total of twelve clinical specialist services offered by this trust that required intensive care support. Through the 18 beds on this site, a total of 1,550 patients per year were managed. This was a large and busy unit that brought with it its own challenges and specific needs.

As a result of the significant levels of activity, bed pressures on this unit were very high. Such pressures were driven by within and outside hospital referrals. In addition, the admission policy of the unit actively encouraged acceptance of patients into the unit at all times. This was reflected in the local unit admission policy that had been supported by both senior nursing and medical staff. The aim was for intensive care patients on this unit to receive a minimum of one to one nursing care, whereas one nurse cared for two high dependency patients. However, due to the need to cover the satellite unit and manage complex patient moves into, and out of the unit, there were times when it was difficult to maintain these ratios without heavy reliance on agency staff.

The unit had a complement of over one hundred nursing staff managed by ten G grade sisters. These staff were then subsequently organised into one of five nursing teams that were each managed by one of the sister group. The nurse specialist/lead nurse and nurse manager led the nursing team. In order to keep the beds at optimal staffing, the recruitment process appeared to be continuous. At the time of the study, the site was starting to experience problems with recruiting experienced critical care nurses and therefore more junior and inexperience staff were being employed. This is now a common experience throughout the intensive care milieu. As a result there was a real commitment and support to junior staff and in-depth induction and orientation programmes were in place. A small team of unqualified and administrative staff supported the running of the unit.

The nursing philosophy of the unit acknowledged 'team co-operation . . . in attaining the highest attainable level of health' and identified the team as the 'greatest resource'. The medical team comprised seven consultant intensivists and physicians who led a team of junior and senior registrars. Different consultants had particular areas of expertise that would be referred to if there was a specific patient problem. In such a large consultant team, it could be six weeks between their on-call weeks on the unit. In addition, the clinical team was complemented by a strong microbiology service and received pharmacy, dietician and physiotherapy support.

Due to the size of the unit and the workforce necessary to service this, there were occasions where nursing staff had not met, and therefore did not know, the capabilities of staff on shift. However, it was evident that the more senior nursing and medical staff had worked alongside each other for some years. Between this group there was an obvious knowledge of each other and their preferred working styles. In their own way, each member of this team showed respect and acknowledged each others' skills and talents in their respective roles.

The unit was focused on the provision of high-quality, research-based care, and primary team nursing had recently been introduced. This differs from primary nursing in that each patient is cared for by a dedicated team of nurses who will care for that patient throughout their stay in intensive care. Communication is passed along that team and each member of that team takes responsibility for progressing that patient's treatment. This unit strongly and actively supported education through nurses attending study opportunities. In addition, there was a well-developed and recognised research expertise in the senior nurses. In-service educational programmes developed by the lead nurse and the newly created lecturer-practitioner also maintained this philosophy.

Nursing interest groups had developed within this unit to explore specific clinical and professional interest areas, for example, use of non-invasive ventilation. One of the on-going projects of specific interest to this research was the development of nursing presentation on the ward round. This had been a project on the unit over the past months and had received mixed response from medical and nursing staff.

Site 2

This site was located in part of a newly refurbished area in a 750-bedded district general hospital. The unit was located away from the other clinical areas, but close to the theatre complex. As the unit had been recently refurbished, it was clean, modern, light and airy for staff and relatives.

Organisationally speaking, the unit was located within the anaesthetics/ theatres and pharmacy directorate of the trust, one of seven clinical directorates. In this directorate there were six other speciality services including theatres, the acute pain clinic and sterile supplies. A director of ICU (consultant) and a senior clinical nurse (nurse manager) led the intensive care unit. It was clear that this director and senior clinical nurse had a strong and developed working relationship that had evolved over the years they had worked together. As opposed to the other sites, there was no specific general manager allocated to the unit *per se*, instead management support was given through the post of the Directorate Manager who oversaw the total anaesthetic directorate.

The unit had six intensive care beds including two side rooms. At the time of the research only five of these beds were operational due to recruitment and funding problems. The unit was geographically and organisationally located adjoining the eight-bedded coronary care unit with the majority of the nursing staff rotating between the two units. The unit had cared for 422 patients during the previous year. Similar to the other sites in this study, the majority of the patients on this unit required admission after elective and emergency surgery. Just under 25 per cent of the patients in this unit were medical patients. Such patients may present with a multiplicity of serious illnesses including those with pneumonia, asthma, those who have taken an overdose, or those who have sustained severe cerebral bleeds. Only a small number of paediatric patients were cared for on the unit with referrals made to the nearby tertiary paediatric centre. On this unit, intensive care patients received a minimum of one-to-one nursing care, but in times of staff shortages combined with bed pressures, the nurse in charge often cared for a patient. On some occasions the ratio was of one nurse to two patients.

The unit had a complement of thirty nursing staff that was organised into three nursing teams. A team of senior nurses including a senior nurse, lecturer practitioner and sister led the nursing team. The team here, although small, was friendly and a stable part of the workforce. The majority of the nursing team had clearly worked together for a number of years. There was a rapport and spirit of team work that was generally evident in all aspects of the work. It was clear that there were motivated individuals who led and nurtured the team on this site. Clinical protocols were being developed and there was evidence of a substantial amount of project work. The medical team comprised three consultant intensivists who lead a team of junior and senior registrars. Again, the nursing team could identify each of the consultants as holding specific interest areas. The sense of commitment to the unit was strong. As the consultant team was only three in number, staff saw them more frequently on the unit. As theatres were nearby, even when not on call for the unit, the consultants popped in to chat with staff. The unit was also strongly serviced by physiotherapy with specific pharmacy support.

An explicit aim of the unit was to provide high quality care. This included recognising and attending to the physical and psychological needs of the individual and his/her carers. This was articulated through the unit philosophy, and enabled through the named nurse concept and the practice of team nursing. This was a further variation on the models of care adopted in the other units. There was evidence of real commitment from the nursing staff to develop protocols for specific aspects of care. Support for staff was equally an important issue on this unit. As well as the well-developed orientation programmes, there were also regular counselling sessions for staff to de-brief on previous distressing clinical incidents. These were offered as interdisciplinary events, but this opportunity was most utilised by the nursing staff.

A further on-going project of specific interest to this research was the establishment and promotion of interdisciplinary meetings including medical, nursing, physiotherapy and management staff. This had been an initiative that had been outlined in a recent business plan. The introduction of such regular meetings was just being established as fieldwork occurred in this site.

Site 3

This site was a Nursing Development Unit (NDU) and located in a purpose-built, modern, 580-bedded hospital. The whole hospital site had been designed with considerable thought; it was light and airy, with a strong use of art throughout the building. Patient information leaflets about the hospital and forms for feedback on hospital performance were readily available in public places.

The organisational structure of the trust was large and complex. Organisationally, the intensive care unit was located within the anaesthetic and imaging clinical directorate; one of the trust's eleven major directorates. Within the anaesthetic directorate, there were a further eleven clinical specialities. These ranged from direct clinical services including intensive care and day care through to investigative services, including an endoscopy suite and support services including sterile supplies. The management team of the intensive care comprised the director of ICU (consultant), operational manager (nurse manager) and clinical nurse specialist/project leader (nurse). This team led clinical unit management.

The ICU was located in one wing of the hospital. It was away from the main ward areas, but located next to the theatre suite. As with the other sites, the doors of the unit were secured. Staff gained entry through knowing the combination for access and visitors used an intercom system to talk to staff who then opened the front doors of the unit. As the unit was purpose built, facilities for staff and relatives were comfortable compared to the other field sites. The unit itself was bright and airy. Natural light and far reaching views out of the windows gave the impression of an agreeable working environment for staff, and of a not too overbearing environment for visitors.

The ICU comprised six intensive care beds (including one isolation room) and four high dependency beds. Two of these HDU beds were operational at the time of the study. The unit cared for any patient in the hospital requiring admission ICU. Over a period of one year, five hundred patients were cared for on this unit. The majority of the patients on the unit were there for support and treatment after elective (routine) and emergency surgery. Such patients comprised nearly 75 per cent of this unit's workload. Patients who undergo major routine surgery may require post-operative ventilation or more intensive monitoring for a short period of time. This particularly occurs if the person has pre-existing cardiac or respiratory disease or if emergency surgical intervention has been required. The remainder of the unit's workload came from patients who had medical problems and required intensive support and treatment. Consistent with health policy in the mid-1990s that led to centralisation of paediatric services, this was not a recognised referral centre for children and so only a small number of children were managed here.

The espoused ethos of this unit was of a strong team approach to care. The unit was well organised and all its senior staff were committed to delivering a quality service. The senior members of the clinical team were a strong and credible force. The senior medical and nursing staff had clearly worked with each other over a prolonged period of time and the respect that they held for each other was very evident. The nursing and medical staff had supported each other and had developed strong working relationships. The influential nursing leaders of this unit had clearly influenced this, both in the past and present. In addition, it appeared that the nursing team was strongly supported by the executive level nurse leaders including the Assistant Director of Nursing and Director of Nursing. Both articulated a strongly patient focused view on how the trust delivered its services.

The unit was well resourced in terms of staffing. It had a complement of over fifty nursing staff, organised into seven primary nursing teams, each led by a team co-ordinator. A clinical nurse specialist and nurse manager led the nursing team, and the philosophy of the unit valued a participatory non-hierarchical management style. This was not just evident in the rhetoric of the unit. This unit demonstrated a real commitment to enable each person to contribute to patient and unit management. On this unit, each intensive care patient was cared for by one nurse per shift. In the high dependency beds, the ratio was of one nurse to two patients. At the time of this research, the use of agency and bank staff was minimal. Support and administrative staff assisted in the daily running of the unit. Recruitment was unproblematic, and retention of staff was not a problem.

The medical team comprised four consultant intensivists who led a team of junior and senior registrars. At the time of the study, all medical staff who rotated through this unit were anaesthetic trainees. The new training programmes for medical staff had not impacted yet and therefore there had been no influx of junior surgeons or physicians. Each consultant was identified as having his or her own area of interest and expertise, and were well spoken of by all staff. The nursing staff noted that some of the consultants had a higher presence on the unit than others and were therefore perceived to be more supportive of the unit. Other key members of this team included the pharmacy, physiotherapy and microbiology support staff who were frequently seen on the unit, and were an intrinsic part of the unit meetings.

A key focus for this unit was the provision of family-centred care as articulated through the nursing philosophy. This was achieved through the practice of primary nursing; this concept was completely embraced by both medical and nursing staff. The overwhelming impression on this unit was the strong culture of development of nurses and of nursing practice. Each of the nursing teams had their own interest areas that developed specific aspects of care given to patients. This activity encouraged involvement of any grade of staff within the flattened organisational structure that existed.

At the time of the study there were some specific on-going projects of interest. The first area I particularly explored was the 'multi-disciplinary meeting'. This was a recurrent issue when staff began to speak about doctors and nurses working together. The second area was the discussion of introducing the clinical governance strategy. The observations made on the differential roles adopted by medicine and nursing within this process was illuminating. Finally, towards the end of the fieldwork, the concept of nursing diagnosis was being initiated trust wide. This again provided an interesting backdrop to explore the introduction of such a uniprofessional concept into an espoused interdisciplinary environment.

The overall impression from this unit was that staff felt supported here and enjoyed working as part of a team. They believed in what they could offer to patients and in how they could make a difference. Staff were welcoming and supportive to all, and were willing to tackle and address issues together. However, it must be noted that substantial investment had gone into this unit. The physical environment within which staff worked was pleasant and the nursing team had received considerable development in terms of nurturing the NDU concept and the nursing staff themselves.

Clinical decision making in context

The purpose of this section is to orientate the reader to where decision making occurred in the clinical context. Through this, it is possible to understand what the key decision-making areas were, and how these areas were developed in intensive care. As the focus of this book is on how doctor and nurses work to make clinical decisions, it is therefore interdependent decision making that is the focus of this chapter.

For me, there were two key areas of clinical decision making by doctors and nurses. These were areas where decisions were made about the patient's clinical management, and those forums that enabled decisions to be made about the clinical service. These are central to this book and are now reviewed in more depth.

The clinical decision-making stage: patient management

There were many discussions between doctors and nurses concerning specific clinical management and treatment issues. The agreed purpose of such discussions was to enable decisions to be made to progress patients' treatment. This may involve discussing the futility of continuing treatment and therefore discussing achieving a peaceful and dignified death for the patient. There were both formal and informal forums for decision making between nurses and doctors. In all the units, discussions about the patient management occurred within the clinical area, either at or close to the patient's bedside. For discussions occurring at the bedside, personnel often gathered around the patent's chart, or at the end of the patient's bed in a semi-circle.

In all sites there were clinical meetings that occurred at relatively set times during the day. Most sites had formal ward rounds twice a day, in the morning and during the afternoon. This event was the ward round. There was a formal structure and set of roles within this forum. The membership of this forum could be large, with a membership that varied from three in the smallest site to fifteen in the largest site. A consultant mainly led the ward rounds, although in their absence the most experienced doctor deputised. The members of the group who were always present for the ward round included the consultant who was in charge on the unit at that time, and the junior doctor(s) covering the unit. The nurse looking after the patient was also usually present, although if the nurse was busy or on break, the ward round continued with just medical members of the team.

The presence of the nurse in charge of the shift was more variable and dependent on unit demands. If there were staff shortages or operational issues to be resolved, the nurse in charge prioritised their workload and attended the round, as he or she was able. The nurse in charge often targeted patients that they wanted to attend the round for. For example, if there was a particularly sick patient requiring decisions to be made or a junior member of staff requiring support, they ensured that they could be present for those particular discussions. In many ways, the ward round was a very egalitarian event. Any grade of nurse or doctor could attend on the ward round, and potentially had the opportunity to participate in patient management decisions. Other disciplines involved in the ward round included physiotherapists, dieticians and microbiologists. Although, these personnel left if the round impinged on patient treatments or other work commitments. This was particularly noticeable in the largest site. With eighteen patients on this site, the ward round could take up to three hours.

In all sites, the ward rounds on Monday mornings were particularly lengthy. The consultant cover for the unit changed on this day and this required all patients to be presented afresh. Conversely, the weekend rounds were noticeably shorter, generally less structured with fewer staff attending. The ward round started in one place and then moved around the unit. In general, patients requiring more immediate treatment decisions were seen first. Patients with an infectious risk were generally seen last, to reduce the risk of cross-infection. The ward round began with the arrival of the consultant and concluded when the medical staff left the unit. The presence of the medical staff was the key factor in determining the ward round. Nursing, physiotherapy and microbiology staff could leave the ward round, but the round continued, even if only medical staff were there. Conversely, if medical staff were called to an emergency, the ward round was terminated.

The process used to develop patient management decisions had a common structure. A problem-focused physiological systems approach was taken across all the sites. This was usually initiated through the junior doctor reviewing the patient's presentation, medical history, particular problems and key events during the intensive care stay. The consultant usually sought further information from the junior doctor, and only occasionally from the nurse. Treatment for the day was then planned. The discussion for that patient was generally concluded with the consultant asking the nurse at the bedside if there were any outstanding issues. This can be seen in the following field notes extract:

> The ward round began when the consultant arrived on the unit, the presence of the nurse in charge was rather haphazard rather than sought. The structure of the ward round began with an in-depth review of the patient using a biomedical model by the junior anaesthetist, this was problem oriented and in priority. There was input from the attending microbiologist with detailed discussion regarding the micro[biology] results and appropriate antibiotic cover. At times this led to break-up discussions with two or three discussions at the same time. This occasionally involved the nurse when issues needed to be clarified or if the nurse informed the team of treatment changes since the last medical review had occurred. After this there appeared to be some general discussion regarding the treatment plan for the next few hours. At the end of the ward round, the consultant turned to the nurse and asked if there were any further issues.

The round then left that patient to move to the next. Once the final patient had been seen, there was sometimes discussion as to the bed state or some general banter between the medical and nursing staff. The round then disbanded.

These formal, predictable patient management forums contrasted with the informal, opportunistic meetings, usually between the nurse at the bedside and the doctor. Informal patient management did not have such defined structure or roles, and was often prompted by a particular or immediate patient problem. Such discussions did not usually include the consultant of the unit unless a particularly complex and critical issue was being discussed, but more frequently occurred with more junior grade medical staff and the nurse at the bedside.

Whilst it appeared that formal and informal patient management forums were distinct, there were connections. Specific patient problems raised in the informal arena were also discussed in the formal ward round. This occurred if the patient problem was significant, or if some dissension had occurred over the decision made in the informal decision-making discussions. In this way the formal ward round was seen as an arbitrator for the decisions made. Key clinical decisions were therefore made in the formal round, and then used to inform, and be informed by the informal decisions made.

The clinical decision-making stage: service management

The second area of decision making in the clinical setting concerned forums used to develop service management decisions. Across the sites, a diverse range of meetings was identified for this purpose. These forums focused on the business or operational management of the clinical unit; either as a discrete unit or as part of the wider trust structure. The forums ranged from local unit meetings with nursing or unit staff to trust level executive meetings and the hospital board. There were meetings that were concerned with general unit management; key operational business issues (service contract meetings); team development (interdisciplinary meetings); trust service planning (strategic planning); and trust specific projects (quality monitoring).

In all sites there were regular management meetings to discuss the clinical service being provided by the unit. Key agenda items included performance on service contracts, unit activity, and personnel or resource issues. Such meetings also acted as a conduit for information from trust management and requests for reports to the trust. Key members of the unit management team (senior nurse, consultant and manager) primarily participated in this area of decision making and the medical director or manager usually chaired such meetings. Accountants and pharmacists attended these meetings to report on expenditure on the unit. The frequency and formality of service management meetings varied across the sites. In all sites, the use of unplanned spontaneous meetings (corridor meetings) were identified as a valuable means of developing unit service management.

All sites held interdisciplinary meetings where any member of the unit team could come to discuss wider clinical unit issues. Attendance at such forums was variable as staff had competing clinical needs to attend to. Medical and nursing attendance was notably sporadic. Nursing staff identified that only those consultants who were the most committed to the unit attended, and consultant staff commented on how nurses would not attend if the meetings were scheduled after their shift had finished. When these forums were scheduled, the agenda items mainly focused on resolution of clinical problems (for example, management of long-term patients) or further dissemination of key management information (for example, cost savings to be made).

There were also uniprofessional meetings that were used to develop specific professional perspectives on unit issues. These were then used to inform management agenda items, both at unit and trust level. Such meetings included medical staff discussing future research and development opportunities, or nursing staff developing specific aspects of care (including improving services for relatives) that were then fed into the broader unit management discussions. With such large nursing workforces, there were regular meetings between the senior nurses and nursing teams to channel information from the trust to all staff. Such meetings also gave opportunity for staff to respond and enable their views to be built into wider unit issues.

The medical staff did not have such an infrastructure on the units. Meetings amongst the medical staff were either held informally amongst the consultants or for junior medical staff, meetings only occurred if specific teaching sessions were held. As most of the junior medical staff were on the units for 2–3 months, they were transient members of the team and were therefore not directly involved in service management.

Involvement in service management issues concerned mainly senior medical, managerial and nursing staff. The forums that enabled decisions to be made in this area were not so formally structured as in forums for clinical decision making. Within the service management arena, the meetings were open to all staff and discussion was encouraged. However, the main agendas were set and upheld by the managerial team. Although there was discussion on improving quality and conditions for care and working, the main areas of debate focused on the financial and activity performance of the clinical units.

What I felt most noticeable was how the three units, although dissimilar in terms of physical environment, capacity offered and some services delivered, did hold great similarity with regards to the culture of support, communication, education and development. All units showed a consistency in personnel who were key to the clinical team, for example, medical, nursing, physiotherapy, and health care scientists. The general working relationships across all sites were very positive, and medical and nursing staff who had worked together for some time had great respect and regard for each other. From this perspective, it appeared that there were harmonious clinical teams in all the units.

Chapter 6

Clinical decision making and the hierarchies of knowledge

In this chapter I explore the main areas of knowledge that were used in decision making in intensive care. From the outset of the fieldwork, it was clear that doctors and nurses used some shared and some distinct types of knowledge to inform patient and service management decisions. To illustrate the results presented, data excerpts are used. Field data appears in quotation marks or in displayed text. Any particular emphasis made by the participants is demonstrated through italic text. Clarification of any abbreviations or terms used by participants is in brackets [ ] in the field data. This format is similarly used through the remaining chapters in this book.

Knowledge used by all clinicians in intensive care was primarily related to the treatment and support of the critically ill patient. This required knowledge of the patient's underlying disease process; an understanding of the potential clinical sequelae; and the specific monitoring and interventions required. There were key areas of knowledge that were familiar to, and used by both doctors and nurses as they worked to support critically ill patients. There were other discrete areas of knowledge that lay principally within, and were used by one discipline.

In the area of clinical service management, the pattern was similar in that both shared and discrete sources of knowledge were revealed. To facilitate effective management of the clinical service, distinct knowledge was used to understand the organisational needs of intensive care; the resources required to provide and sustain the service; and how to work within the systems required to support service delivery. There were well defined areas that were monitored and reported on in order to maintain the health of the service. These were key areas of knowledge that were recognised and used by the clinical management team (doctors, nurses and managers) as they worked to manage the units. Some knowledge was shared and used by doctors, nurses and managers but there were other discrete areas of knowledge that were only held and used by one discipline. In this way, the clinical and service management fields demonstrated two very different, and yet parallel worlds.

This chapter will explore the shared and the distinct areas of knowledge used in clinical and service management decisions. The importance of the objective, scientific model in decision making will be demonstrated. The marginalisation of holistic knowledge of the patient and family, and the importance of ethical care and provision of physical comfort in intensive care are explored. Through drawing attention to the importance attached to specific areas of knowledge, and the devaluation of other areas of knowledge, I will demonstrate the existence of a hierarchy of knowledge in decision making.

Areas of knowledge: the shared and the discrete

As highlighted in the introductory paragraphs, when making decisions in intensive care, specific domains of knowledge were used to direct discussion and debate. In clinical patient management, scientific, biomedical information was the most frequently used source of knowledge by doctors and nurses. This knowledge base encompassed anatomical, physiological and biochemical knowledge and was used to underpin the understanding of therapies used in critical illness. All doctors and nurses used such knowledge in making decisions about clinical management, as this excerpt demonstrates:

> Doctor: So how's it going here? Nurse: Well, let's see, resp [respiratory] wise we're fully ventilated and on high FIO_2. She's still desaturating on turning, so we're hyperoxygenating her. Cardiovascular, well she's on Norad. with mean arterial pressures of 70. We're volume loading her, and her acidosis is worsening. What parameters are we working towards? – I'm sure she's overloaded. Anyhow, her last urine was 20mls this hour.

In the ward round, this biomedical knowledge was used in the majority of discussions. My field journal notes: 'The focus on the ward round is very scientifically focused. There are discussions about biochemistry, labs [laboratory] tests. There is much discussion about cause of the patient's problem, other treatment options, what physiological parameters are to be aimed for.'

As described in Chapter 5, discussions on the ward round were inevitably initiated by a patient problem, to which a treatment solution was offered, and its effectiveness evaluated using key physiological parameters. This gave rise to the standard approach taken during discussion of patient problems either during the ward round, or informally at the bedside. As described by one doctor: 'The problems are presented. It is up to me to put forward the treatment plan and then review it on the next round. Nurses ask for fixed evaluation points to help manage the problem – especially with haemodynamics.'

The prevalence of the biomedical model in intensive care was evident. It gave structure to patient presentation and management in the ward round and during medical and nursing handovers, and was used to systematically order entries in both medical and nursing notes. It was the area of knowledge shared by medicine and nursing and was the focus of the joint problem solving. Examination of the nursing documentation revealed a use of the biomedical model with key physiological systems worked through, and then with specific areas of nursing knowledge added on at the end. The particular areas attributed to nursing were not formally presented or discussed with medical staff. As a result, doctors perceived health care knowledge to reflect predominantly medical knowledge. The biomedical model was perceived therefore to be the model of medicine and not a model used and shared by nursing and medicine.

Although both medical and nursing staff used this scientific knowledge, discussion of it lay primarily in the domain of medicine. The educational preparation of medical staff provided doctors with a more in-depth scientific awareness, but nurses also had appreciation of this area. Despite the fact that nurses used such knowledge to underpin their thought processes in patient assessment and interventions, nurses rarely demonstrated their possession of it in decision-making forums. It was clear that, in intensive care, the dominant knowledge base used in the decision-making process was held, and directed by medicine. As highlighted by Fox (1993), it appeared that this was sustained through the ability of medical staff to control the ward round agenda.

This dominant position of medical knowledge in defining illness and treatment in health care has been well explored in the sociological literature (Freidson 1994). Through use of the biomedical framework, medicine demonstrates an established authority (Netherton 1995). In this, patients become anonymous, depersonalised and passive beings (Sinclair 1997) and reframed as diagnosis and treatments (Busby and Gilchrist 1992). This was demonstrated in the ward rounds when complete discussions occurred around, for example, potassium losses and organ perfusion pressures. As identified by Lawler (1997) this led to the reporting of the body often being undertaken in a depersonalised manner, rendering the body theoretically and epistemologically fragmented.

Medical authority in decision making was demonstrated through an apparent hierarchy existing within the areas of clinical knowledge used in intensive care. This was most frequently evidenced with topics perceived to be nursing knowledge. As noted by one doctor: There are certain areas in the ward round that I bequeath to nursing – the choice of beds, those clinically superficial areas – bowel care, skin care, mouth care, wound care.' The use of the term 'clinically superficial' was used here to illustrate those areas supposed by medical staff to have less impact on the clinical management of the patient. Such areas as bowel care and skin care were therefore of less concern and less importance to medicine. These areas were infrequently discussed as part of the recognised ward round agenda. The use of the word 'bequeathing' intimates power and authority to assign areas to the domain of others.

The method by which knowledge gained credibility in this hierarchy was revealing. This is perhaps best illustrated through a medical reaction in one unit to a nursing interest in complementary therapy, described as the 'touchy feely side of nursing' by one medical consultant. I asked the nurse if she could explain this some more: 'It's his little logo, but just some of the nursing staff have got very strong interests in alternative therapies . . . he will not entertain the idea of aromatherapy at all, he lacks support for it.' The issue of interest here is not about one individual's decision to support or not support a therapy. The decision was based on the lack of credibility that aromatherapy possessed within the medical knowledge framework. It had therefore been labelled as 'touchy feely', a descriptor not associated with the scientific model of medicine. As it did not have the support of medicine, it was not used on this unit.

In service management there were also specific areas that had been informally organised into a structure to direct debate and discussion in clinical directorate meetings. These areas included activity monitoring, budgetary expenditure and contractual arrangements, and they required knowledge of the intensive care therapy service. A hierarchy of knowledge existed in this domain. When determining the service agenda, economic and financial knowledge held the greatest importance. As this doctor states:

> the financial squeeze makes decisions difficult, the humanist point of view just doesn't work on the floor. Money is the catalyst. We can now charge user directorates on a fee for basis. We are cost conscious here and try to drive costs down. Money should buy personnel and equipment . . . We would support directorates as long as there was a cost neutral effect.

Any issues, specifically any nursing issues, not related directly to finance were poorly acknowledged or supported in service forums:

> It is usually difficult to get nursing issues on to these agendas. For example, it has been difficult to get a bereavement counsellor on the unit. It is only after the ICS [Intensive Care Society] had issued guidelines that it got taken seriously by the medical staff.

A higher priority status was therefore afforded to certain areas of knowledge, and a valid place on the decision-making agenda was gained if associated financial implications were identified, or unless there was support from medicine. Senior nurses were aware of this and they developed strategies to get their areas of concern onto the management agenda. Through articulating the financial implications of the problem or proposal, nursing issues could find a place on the service management agenda. In this excerpt, a nurse speaks about obtaining support for clinical supervision:

> Clinical supervision is going to be costly – initially it was just a nursey thing, but then when we costed it out and they realised that it was going to cost £12–13K there were problems. But we constructed our arguments about recruitment and retention, a real problem for us, then they went with it. If it had no impact in finances or their role, it would have been left as a nursing thing.

The nursing knowledge used in service decisions was therefore restricted to discussion under financial issues. In accord with Traynor's findings (1996), the concepts and methods of the marketplace had been adopted in service management decision making. The key agenda items where nursing was discussed therefore related to staffing costs, skill mix and opening of beds. In this way, financial knowledge was used as a means of inspection of, and control, over nursing. Service knowledge possessed by nurses did not appear to exist outside these areas. Other areas of nursing knowledge achieved only a token presence, found within the rhetoric of quality care and best practice issues. Whilst medicine in service management was similarly governed by a financial discourse; the difference was in the degree of impact. In service management, medical staff continued to have the freedom and autonomy to practise with few limitations: nursing was more restricted and restrained by the dominance of management knowledge and agendas.

Bigger or peripheral issues?

As demonstrated in the previous section, there were areas of knowledge used to inform clinical and service delivery issues that were not shared by all. These areas were reflective of the previously referred to as 'clinically superficial'. One nurse reflected: 'I think the issues that doctors immediately think of when nurses raise issues are wound care, relatives, rashes, pressure areas.' Such areas of knowledge were all readily identifiable in nursing practices and as part of the framework in the nursing documentation. Both doctors and nurses highlighted the effect that experience and training had on the use of this knowledge in the process of decision making. As discussed by this doctor:

> The distance between doctors and nurses has narrowed as nurses are more knowledgeable . . . the D and junior E grade staff nurses are like very junior registrars. They raise issues about what shall we do about the feed, the antibiotics. The more experienced the nurses are, the more questions they will raise. The more senior nurses will raise questions like – what are we doing here? And sometimes they raise it too much [laughs]. What should we be doing about the family? – particularly when dealing with planning a difficult game plan.

As a result of this common understanding of what doctors perceived to be nursing issues on the ward round, these areas of nursing knowledge were regarded as being on the 'periphery' of clinical decision making by medical staff. Such issues were therefore poorly recognised, if at all. This often resulted in the ward round being dominated by medical discussion. Only at the end was the nurse consulted:

> At the end of one patient discussion when the nurse had been standing in the circle, the patient needed attending to and the nurse had to turn her

back to see the patient. When she turned back, the team was walking away, without asking her if any issues were to be raised. She called after them: *Excuse me.* It was only after the third attempt that she succeeded in calling them back. They apologised and she then asked her questions regarding the patient's management.

In the study undertaken by Manias and Street (2001b), nurses themselves recognised that their concerns got 'tagged on to the end'. In their study, this actually gave rise to nurses in one unit calling themselves the TAG team. Medical staff felt that nursing issues were on the fringes of medical treatment and care, but for nurses themselves such issues were intrinsic to their knowledge base and skills and therefore were seen to be part of a larger, more expanded knowledge base required for the total management of the critically ill patient. Nurses therefore perceived these areas to contribute to the 'bigger picture' of the decision making and felt medicine ignored and devalued their expertise and their concerns.

The language of knowledge

Medical staff asserted that use of a biomedical, scientific knowledge base led to providing rational, objective measurements:

> Nurses need to be more specific. Like on the ward round I go round and they say 'we had to put the pressure support up' and I ask why. He was tired is what they say. And I ask 'What do you mean by that? I'm looking for objectivity, for an increased respiratory rate – *start to talk about things you can measure.*

Calculable variables, the use of quantitative data, were seen by medicine to be more robust than qualitative data. This ethos was shared within the service management arena. The following excerpt is from an interview with a doctor. In it he had been discussing nurse staffing in intensive care:

> Regarding one-to-one care, I think that it is important to demonstrate safety – but you can't prove it – a lot of it is based on arguments about quality. *But does inventing a new language help?* Quantitative arguments are difficult to overturn. *Hard facts are visible – patient mortality is measurable.*

As a result, medical staff were frustrated with the inability of nurses to defend their arguments on the clinical ward round. This next excerpt is illustrative of this:

> On the ward round, one nurse asks about pre-oxygenating before suctioning a sick patient. The doctor asks why this should be necessary. The

nurse replies: because he takes a long time to recover. Doctor: How long? Nurse: Well, I haven't exactly seen it drop myself. The doctor then asks who has seen it drop and the nurse replies that the night staff have seen it. The doctor, then, looking straight at me says: well how *far* did it drop? The nurse replies: 87 per cent. Doctor: Don't worry then.

During my interview with the doctor later on that morning, this incident was again raised: 'Just look at what happened on the ward round. I ask for clarification and what I get is "Well that is what is handed over to me". *For God's sake*, they're capable of thinking.' Without exception, the language used by nurses to articulate their knowledge provoked extraordinarily strong comments from the medical staff in this study:

> Nurses use their own language – like models. Nurses just collect a bit of evidence and then walk away. They can just *bellyache*. Look at the language they use. I think they ought to get rid of the RCN [Royal College of Nursing] and the patient needs of elimination. *Too much emphasis on number one.*

It was clear that medical staff and general managers uniformly supported the superiority of numerical data and rational, objective thought. This left an impression of medicine and management being rigorous, evidenced-based and reliable. However, there were staff who questioned the reality of this in the intensive care environment. As one doctor highlighted: 'It is difficult in ICU because there is little hard evidence. It is impossible to do a random control group test with a heterogeneous group.' This lack of research was cited as causing further problems. One junior doctor commented: 'I think one problem about intensive care medicine is the lack of research in the area. This leads to different management styles in patient treatment as no one is really sure of the answer.'

This situation particularly impacted on the diverse ways of managing particular patient problems within the units. Nurses and junior doctors noted this variability in clinical practice, especially in the practice of unit consultants. Variations in management were particularly noticeable to nursing staff as they had direct contact with all the medical consultants: 'Nurses see a greater difference between consultants – they [the consultants] don't believe them when you tell them.' Others in the medical team also experienced the impact of these changes. As identified by one senior registrar: 'Every time the medical consultant changes, for example with the weaning, some will say, wean down on the pressure support or some will say take the patient off for an hour every day. I think it doesn't really matter – just be consistent.'

The alteration in treatment was noticeable when consultants changed from one week to another and particularly noticeable in certain practices, for example ventilator preferences, the type of invasive monitoring, specific use of drugs. However, as consultants did not overlap or work with each other, they did not identify this as a problem. If the medical staff did acknowledge concerns existed, these were rationalised:

> I think we all agree on the major changes – on directions of treatment and so on. There may be some minor treatment changes visible and I think that the nurses see those and argue that there is a lack of continuity. I don't make an apology for it. I think that for the week that the medical consultant is on you get total continuity, and I think that it works well.

For medical staff, such issues related to minor treatment changes. For nurses, such treatment changes were the bread and butter of their work. Such continued acceptance of the diversity of approaches to patient management served to re-enforce the authority of medicine. However with the advent of protocolised clinical standards and guidelines, it also raises questions about the legitimacy of medical knowledge.

It was primarily nursing staff who introduced strategies to address such inconsistencies: 'We have changed the structure of the handover on Monday so that it is consultant to consultant as a compromise to try to minimise this effect.' The use of clinical guidelines and protocols had been adopted in another unit to minimise the variance in practice. As outlined by one nurse: 'Guidelines and policies are for practice, for the way that we work. They are to maintain safety. If you look at what happened here with feeding patients – they all wanted different things'. The important issue to note here is that even though this problem lay within the practice of medicine, it was the nursing staff who attempted to gain some consensus; despite the fact that it was an area over which they had little direct authority.

Although discrepancies in medical knowledge and practice have been highlighted in national health policy (Audit Commission 1999), they have received little empirical attention (Hatt 1998). Medical differences in decision making regarding patient management are not universally acknowledged (McKee and Clarke 1995). Nurses often raised the issue amongst themselves that if patient treatment can be measured and articulated in a rational and objective manner as advocated by medicine, then it should appear logical that clinical practice could be standardised. However, as pointed out by one nurse: 'All the clinical policies are discussed, but the doctors still want some room for clinical judgement – yes that's fine they say, but it still needs to go on clinical judgement.'

The concern here may not be about clinical judgement, but about maintaining individual and collective medical autonomy and authority. As has been observed by Liaschenko (1998), nurses in this study noticed the limitations of medical knowledge, and recognised that medicine was not faultless. However, operating at the edge of such competing epistemologies, nurses did not attest to this, and often remained silent (Alavi and Cattoni 1995). Therefore, by this action – or lack of action – medical dominance continued to be uncontested.

Knowing the whole

In intensive care, the critical nature of the patient illness led to a high family presence in the unit. The nurse caring for the patient spent considerable time supporting the family. When the patient was unconscious, the nurse was able to 'know' the patient as a person through the family. This source of knowledge was not completely unique to nursing, but was more developed by nurses. One doctor commented that: 'Nurses are with the patient for 24 hours a day on a one-to-one level. A lot are very emotionally involved and get to know the family – medical staff do as well. It's just that it takes a little longer.'

This source of knowledge was routinely used in the nursing handover in every site. This excerpt from shift handover is an example:

> The nurse then gives details of patient name, age and important issues in medical history. A review of the key problems over the patient's stay and a more detailed account of the previous shift is given . . . The patient's family are mentioned unless the patient is short stay [i.e. overnight surgical patient] or there are problem issues: I'll hand over the details to whoever takes over. The final issue covered is the patient team and the patient's primary nurse . . . The group [oncoming shift] walk around the unit stopping at the end of each bed listening to the report, unless there is something sensitive i.e. information regarding a [patient] deterioration when families are present.

Knowledge about the person and family was seen to be an important source of data to inform patient management. As one nurse commented: 'What do I think that the nurse's greatest contribution to the ward round is? – Well, I think that they can contribute the most in terms of updating and providing information on the patient and their relatives – on the emotional side regarding the family.'

This aspect of knowing the whole, of knowing the patient and family, was a central part of the nursing philosophy at both local unit and trust level. It was an explicit part of the nursing documentation and evident in details recorded about the social history of the patient, their 'significant others' and any information shared with the family. Across all trust sites, there was evidence of the importance of this focus in local unit projects and information booklets provided by nursing staff for visiting family and friends.

The expanded nursing knowledge of the patient through knowledge of the family is a well recognised central part of the nursing philosophy of caring (Leininger 1985). Concern for the emotional and psychological support of patient and family is reflected in much of nursing's literature (Watson 1979, Benner 1984). Informed by a person–centred approach, the conceptualisation of nursing has developed from physically focused nurse–patient interactions, as described by Macleod-Clark (1983), to delivery of a more purposeful, directive and interpersonal care (Gadow 1985).

Medical staff did not have such a developed concern for this area. This is perhaps best illustrated by the following extract from a nursing and medical handover regarding a nine-month-old baby with severe cerebral palsy. The baby had suffered from recent cerebral bleeds, resulting in brain damage. The decision had been made to offer supportive treatment only. In the nursing report there were lengthy details of how staff lived in the same village, and how they had christened the child on the unit, with staff acting as godparents.

> · Handover from nurse in charge: 'As a result it's a one-way wean. We are preparing for extubation. No one knows how he'll do so we are preparing the family. Alice [the nurse] knows the family and would like to stay'. The nursing staff in report are quiet, avoid eye contact with each other for a few seconds. Then express concern over the next few minutes. Comments such as 'how awful', 'that poor family'.

> The same baby is handed over in a medical report: Nine-month-old cerebral palsy with numerous cerebral infarcts, for a one-way wean and all that tragic stuff – plan to extubate and see how we go. Not for further intervention. No further comment was passed by either doctor. The next patient on the unit was then immediately discussed.

The medical handover was short and factual. No details were discussed regarding the support required by or given to the family. I acknowledge that interpersonal and gender issues may have influenced medical staff's engagement in this area. However, the point here is that this area was not one in which medical staff sought knowledge in their handover.

Gaining knowledge of the whole led to the opportunity for nurses to provide emotional support for the whole family unit. As highlighted by this nurse: 'The two [nursing and medicine] are very similar, the key difference is that nursing is very much a day-to-day 24-hour support, knowing the family as a whole, picking up how they are coping and what sort of support networks they have got.' This knowledge was also used to prepare the family for future anticipated problems: 'The nurse will liaise with the family, it is important for them [the family] to know what the medical team are thinking.'

By the very nature of intensive care work, all members of the health care team had interaction with families. Both medical and nursing staff were involved in their support. However, both doctors and nurses saw nurses as possessing a closer focus on this area of knowledge:

> the doctors will say that we get obsessed with the family, and they don't see it as a priority, but when you're with the family for 24 hours, you can see why you have that perspective at the forefront of your mind. I'm not saying that physiological support isn't important.

Families met and spoke with the nurses while visiting their loved one in intensive care. Medical staff spoke to families if changes occurred in the patient's condition, or as prompted by the nursing staff: 'Mrs S.'s family haven't been seen for some time. Could someone see them when they come in?' The practice in all of the units was for a nurse to be present when a doctor spoke to a family. Very often, after a doctor had spoken to the family, the nurse stayed for a while afterwards to ensure that they understood the information given and continue to offer support. The intensive care nurse was part of the technical world of the intensive care unit, but had some comprehension of the world of the family. The nurse therefore mediated between the world of high technological medicine and the human response to illness in the intensive care setting. In this way, one nurse saw her role as being: 'the interface between the patient's family and the hospital system.'

Emotional care and support of the patient and family were important to nurses. Field observation demonstrated that nurses invested much time in this area. Medical staff were not uninformed of the knowledge that nursing staff possessed. However, in terms of giving importance to knowledge of the family and patient, medicine and nursing had different perspectives, as was made explicit by this doctor:

> I mean the nurse come on at 8, they come into the office with their coffee for 'handover' and for allocation – God only knows what they talk about – it's not a handover, it's a chat. They then come out and get a second handover from the patient's nurse, about nursey things, about relatives, not medical things.

Consistent with the literature (Hayes 1990; Curry 1995), the nurses in this study placed great emphasis on the knowledge gained through establishing a relationship with the patient and the family. It is through meeting and managing such needs (Norheim 1989; Busby and Gilchrist 1992) that this discrete source of knowledge in intensive care nursing is acquired.

The general feeling by nurses was that this area of knowledge was not seen to be 'medical' by medicine. The decision-making agenda did not accommodate discussion of these issues and therefore this area of nursing knowledge was poorly utilised. This aspect of knowledge was felt by nurses to be devalued by medicine, to be seen as on the peripheries of decision making, to be hidden. As this nurse asserted:

> I think that the nursing focus is different, nurses focus on pain, relatives, these are the areas they see as important. Doctors see these areas as on the peripheries . . . But doctors don't see the hidden things . . . they only see the visual overt things.

Within the service management arena, a similar knowledge was displayed of knowing the nursing 'family'. The same ethos of interpersonal care was translated throughout the supportive measures undertaken by senior staff. The senior nurses spent considerable amounts of time supporting and talking with the nurses, as individuals and as part of the teams they were organised into for their support. The fundamental nature of the educational programmes offered on the units was underpinned by the espoused principle of development. Again this was an area where skills and investment were required in order to be able to build knowledge; such investment was poorly recognised by managers and medicine and was rarely used as a credible source in service planning. Within a health service driven by strong economic motives, there is increasing risk that such non-quantifiable aspects of nursing practice could be rendered vulnerable (Reeve 1993). Talking with patients or supporting staff may then become no more than just passing the time (Reeve 1993). 'Knowledge of the whole' may therefore be rendered invisible in the systems of workload measurement, ignored by management and medicine, and committed to an 'epistemological silence' (van Maanen 1990, p. 113).

Providing emotional care requires effort, as has been studied through the sociological concept of emotional labour (Hochschild 1983). Emotional labour at work remains invisible (James 1989) and, because of its unquantifiable, essentially feminine characteristics (Phillips 1996), is poorly remunerated. Both doctors and nurses invest emotional labour in intensive care, but in this study it was clear that nurses spent considerably more energy and interest in this area. The emotional labour invested by nurses was spent not only in acting as the main interface for the family in intensive care, but also in working with medicine in negotiating the decision-making process. The emotional labour invested by nurses was not, at any time, acknowledged. Failure to recognise emotional labour in intensive care nursing continues to uphold the hierarchy of traditional knowledge and skills in the delivery of contemporary health care. The broader aspects of nursing knowledge in clinical or management practice continue to be undervalued, and therefore medical hegemony is sustained.

Intensive care not intensive torture

One area of practice where strong concerns were raised by both medical and nursing staff were the ethical perspectives held within the clinical team. The ideology of caring associated with nursing and the close association with, and knowledge of, the patient implicitly places nurses in a position where they are very aware of patient and relative suffering (Soderberg et al. 1997; Schneider 1997; Norrie 1997). In intensive care, this was demonstrated through nursing staff being focused on the need for patient comfort and support. This was central to the knowledge that nurses derived about the critically ill patient and resonated in the very nature of discussions in the clinical field.

Nurses did not believe that doctors, as a group, gave the same emphasis to the need for ethical care. Medical staff were perceived by nurses as continuing to treat patients when nursing staff felt that there was poor prospect of improvement. This is well encapsulated in the following fieldwork entry, made by a nurse:

> Nurses are there to give a reality check, to act as patient advocate, to raise the issues the relatives, or you think the patient would want. We see patients with more dignity. It is meant to be intensive care and not intensive torture. Doctors find it difficult to say 'enough's enough' – they become mixed up with all the technology available, the litigation issues.

The position adopted by all nurses was that the quality of life for the patient was paramount, and should be an explicit part of the knowledge used in clinical management. One nurse commented on the: 'inappropriate management of a 72-year-old man who was kept alive needing increasing amounts of drugs'. She felt that the man should be allowed to die with dignity. This issue was very often closely aligned to the quality of life for relatives with a long-term patient making little progress in intensive care. With patients who had been very sick over a prolonged period of time, nurses started voicing concerns, often in the coffee room first to other colleagues, and then more formally to medical staff regarding patient treatment. The frustrations caused by ethical situations were particularly evident with those patients who had been in the unit for, what nurses considered to be, a long time with little hope of recovery:

> They don't look at the quality issues of life. *I mean, someone in here for 81 days.* That sort of issue should have been addressed ages ago – there are never any case conferences to look at where we are going with the patient, and how things ought to be done.

It was knowledge of the patient and their family that shaped the ethical perspectives held by the nurse. Medical staff were not necessarily privy to such extensive knowledge of the patient and therefore required time to assess the patient using similar benchmarks. This included, for example, how quickly the patient was or was not progressing or understanding the family's views on their loved one's treatment. This 'checking-out' procedure was particularly evident at the beginning of the week when the consultants handed over. The nursing perception across the sites is reflected here: 'You know you're not likely to get a decision on Monday. You may have been struggling all weekend to get some plan for the patient, and then comes Monday.'

However, the ethics of care was clearly a key consideration in medical decision making. There were patients who, during the study, were not admitted into intensive care as medical staff felt that they would not benefit from intensive treatment. Such judgements were often based on subjective perceptions and their previous clinical experiences. The ethics of care for nurses did not appear to hold such an explicit priority in the medical knowledge framework. In the ward rounds, junior medical staff were not likely to raise such issues with consultants and remained silent. This resulted in reliance by some medical staff on nurses: 'Nurses bring up ethical issues – especially if the consultant is rushed.'

As shown in Wicks's work (1998), unless nurses were able to strongly and assertively articulate their position, the medical standpoint inevitably informed clinical decision making. As a result, the medical and nursing ethical positions were not always congruent and led to conflict. Nursing distress in this type of situation has been documented (Fowler 1989). Oberle and Hughes (2001) give an alternative reading to this situation. They suggest that medical and nursing staff may actually hold very similar ethical perspectives. The perceived discrepancies may result from the different professional role functions held by medicine and nursing, and not the different ethical reasoning or moral motivations.

Arising from ethical knowledge was concern for patient comfort. This was a key issue frequently raised by medicine and nursing in clinical forums. As stated earlier, nurses perceived sedation and pain relief as a key component of their role and acted to ensure that their patient was not distressed. This included the administration of sedatives to keep patients settled. However, a different view was often expressed by medicine: 'Nurses want to focus on sedation – they think I don't see it as a problem – it is, but it's much more . . . I'm looking at the plan for the next two days, and if we give the patient more sedation, we won't get them off the ventilator.'

Sedation and analgesia administration were within the remit of the nurse. Once prescribed by the medical staff, drugs were then administered within given parameters (for example, morphine infusion 0–5mg/hr) and increased at the nurse's discretion. With the availability of more sophisticated ventilators and an increase in demand for intensive care, a change in practice has been required to sedate patients lightly and therefore enable quicker weaning times from ventilators. An interesting development in intensive care has been the introduction of objective, numerical scales to monitor and optimise patient sedation. This tool was mentioned in a medical interview: 'Sedation – nurses either do it perfectly, or disastrously. It's in the nurse's control. Using the sedation scale you can see if the sedation needs to be increased or decreased.'

Sedation and pain relief was an issue for both medicine and nursing. However, it was not entirely viewed in the same way by each group and was therefore prioritised differently. The distress felt by nurses from being with a patient in pain or discomfort was exacerbated by the fact that the nurse was constantly at the bedside. Nurses generally believe that: 'for them [doctors] to come in for an hour – it's not the same.' Effective pain relief is consistent with nursing's philosophical beliefs. Medicine perceived that the need for sedation has been driven by a fundamentally subjective nursing assessment, leading to over-sedation of the patient. Scientific rating scales have been introduced to make this area of assessment objective and therefore logical.

This illustrates the different perspectives held by each discipline in this area. Through the responses made to this clinical issue, the measures that doctors and nurses use to maintain control over their respective areas of practice is evident.

The challenge for nurses has been to work with the sedation scales so that they can rationally and articulately defend their clinical decision making. The sedation scales may well have enabled accurate assessment of patient need and thus met medicine's requirements in this area. What has been overlooked are the nursing issues associated with caring for a lightly sedated, intubated patient, or the ability to deliver on the ever-increasing workload at the bedside.

At times, medicine and nursing appear to reflect two competing ethical perspectives. The debate about nursing and medical ethics has been well informed by sociological discussion on the masculine and feminine approaches to ethics (Gilligan 1982, Gallagher 1995). Although such work has been illuminating, a working solution is still required that engages both masculine and feminine ethics within one working environment. The eclectic principle offered by Gillon that 'different voices need to be heard, understood and combined into an adequately complex and mature health care' (1992, p. 172) is attractive, but further work on the pragmatic detail of how this can be attained is still needed.

Knowledge from continuity

It will have been noted from the profiles of the units detailed earlier that there were large numbers of nursing staff working on the units. This was with the aim of achieving the traditionally accepted ratio of one nurse caring for one patient during each shift (British Medical Association 1967). Despite the fact that this has been a contentious issue for some years (Miranda et al. 1997; Pilcher et al. 2001), it was the gold standard that all the units aimed for. This approach led to a constant nursing presence at the bedside 24 hours a day. As one nurse said: 'The nurse is here 24 hours a day – she should know what is happening – there is continuity of care.' In reality of course, this was a collective, rather than an individual presence. No one nurse was on duty for the whole day. Often during that period of time, two or three nurses cared for one patient in shifts.

In order to provide greater continuity to the patient and family, there were certain initiatives that were in place across the units. For example, aspects of care were documented on observation charts and in the patient's notes; including wound care management, communication with the family, and a day activity rota for long-stay patients. Each unit also had locally agreed arrangements to organise nursing working patterns to enhance continuity of care (for example, primary nursing, team nursing). All members of the clinical teams strongly believed in the benefits of such arrangements. As acknowledged by one of the medical staff: 'The concept of team nursing as practised here brings continuity to the care and the experienced nurse can bring insight into what is going on for the patient.'

The continuity of care was derived from the depth of understanding of patient and family needs, and the ability to communicate this to staff on oncoming shifts. This continual presence at the bedside places the nurse in an ideal position to assess and monitor the patient (Davies 1995) and gives rise to a unique source of knowledge. All the medical staff were aware of this: 'The key issue in nursing is that the individual nurse is at the bedside continuously, and therefore they have a better insight into the natural fluctuations of the patient and the family.'

The fact that nurses accessed detailed patient information has been established. What has not been established is how, or if this information was utilised. A frequent topic of conversation in the field was the frustration experienced by nurses who 'knew the patient', and on offering this information to doctors, had this rebuked: 'Why don't they just filter her? We know that in the past she becomes really unstable if her pH drops below 7.3.'

Nurses often found it difficult that their knowledge of the patient was not taken account of and integrated into what was then perceived as medicine's patient management plan. To resolve such situations, there was often a trade-off where nurses rationalised their actions. The following situation illustrates this well:

> The nurse has been asked by the medical consultant to reduce the sedation on the patient. The nurse has looked after this patient for several shifts now. The nurse is obviously very unhappy with this decision, and is verbally and non-verbally indicating that she does not agree with him. Turning to me she talks: The medical consultant wants to assure himself of her neuro. [neurological] status. I've explained to him that she gets uncomfy [uncomfortable], that we have little room for manoeuvre but he wants the sedation reduced. He's usually very good on a one to one, but he wants this. He says we can put it back up but I think she's *so brittle* that we just have *no room* for negotiation. She's on 100 per cent PCV. *Well, I suppose one episode and we'll know.*

Here the nurse attempted to rationalise the treatment action requested through citing the usual good working relationships with the consultant and the ability to review the order if further problems occurred. Although, as an experienced nurse, she had insight into those natural fluctuations referred to, this appeared to be ignored. The point being made here is not about individuals and their responses. As the following excerpt shows, medical staff espouse a commitment to listening and understanding nursing knowledge of the patient: 'Nurses play a key role in the ward round, in assessing the patient, and yet nurses find it difficult to chip in. The registrars don't always present the patient well. Nurses are getting better, but they are frightened – but why? They say – But I'm only a nurse. Yes, but you are there for 24 hours, and I'm only here for 5 minutes and your observational skills are better than mine.' Whilst the discourse of scientific medicine articulates its recognition of the experience of others, the questions of how and if such sources of knowledge are used, are debatable.

Knowledge gained from being a 'continuous' presence on the unit was also displayed in the management of the service. The senior nurses were located on the unit for the majority of their working hours. It therefore fell to them to resolve day-to-day management problems and make decisions about how to manage the discrete areas that were essential for the smooth running of the service. Managing this process can be explored through examining the inter-disciplinary unit meetings held on all the units. There were some medical staff who were committed to a team unit approach and supported such events, but others were noticeable by their absence. To the nurses this represented a lack of commitment to the unit, and a lack of involvement in broader unit activities. One senior nurse commented: 'Well, take patient case conferences or the recent discussion we had on infection control practices, for example. Some [medical staff] will religiously attend and help to uphold what is the agreed. Others don't turn up and then when it's their week on, we have to remind them of what has been agreed.' In this way, the nursing staff provided continuity to sustain the decisions made.

The way that medical work is organised undoubtedly prevents medical staff having the same degree of knowledge of the environment as is held by nursing staff. Temporal and spatial factors affect the nature of medical work (Atkinson 1995). Medical work by the very nature of its organisation cannot routinely build such close working partnerships with patients, families and the unit environment. This situation is understandable. However, the contention is that the knowledge gained from proximity to the clinical and service environment continues to be relegated in a subordinate position to the dominant medical knowledge base.

Knowledge of the environment

There was a final area of knowledge used in clinical decision making that was poorly reflected in interviews, but clearly evident in the field observations. This area was concerned with knowledge used to get things done. A key component of this area concerned how nurses worked with the clinical environment and organisational system to contribute to both patient and service management decisions. As was stated by one consultant: 'The nurse is the key to getting things done, to getting things working properly.'

The subtle but complex activities undertaken by nurses, to ensure the operational running of the total process of care and service delivery, appeared taken for granted in the clinical and organisational setting. Such knowledge remained invisible not only to doctors, but also to nurses. When I discussed this knowledge with medical and nursing staff, it became clear that skills required for example, to prime an infusion set to deliver medication or to manage a staff budget, were just accepted as 'part of the job'. Such activities were not seen as a source of knowledge (Jacques 1993; Liaschensko 1998).

One area where this sort of knowledge was demonstrated well is the use of equipment in intensive care. Intensive care treatment is often mediated through machines. A ventilator gives mechanical support to the breathing of a critically ill patient; infusion pumps regulate drug therapy and pharmacological support to patients; and haemofiltration machines offer mechanical support to the kidneys. The patient's bedside can be surrounded by a plethora of machines. Knowledge is required to work with these machines. For an intensive care clinician, this knowledge becomes familiar territory, and possibly, I would suggest, is internalised as tacit knowledge (Carper 1978). This may account for its relative absence during the interviews, yet being clearly identifiable during the field observations. Although medical staff did alter ventilation settings or infusion pumps settings and some units had technicians to support and trouble-shoot, the nursing staff appeared to be the key workers with the machines at the bedside. As one nurse commented:

> Doctors have a reduced knowledge regarding aspects of the machines. For example, the doctors state 'aim for a zero balance on the haemofiltration'. The nurses set up the machine, operate it, place the patient on/off it, troubleshoot it, etc.

Despite the seminal work of Benner (1984), nurses in this study appeared to devalue their technical knowledge in a clinical world that valued scientific knowledge. The manner in which nurses integrated knowledge gained from the machines and monitors into their worldview was revealing. In one medical interview it was stated: 'here they treat the machines as an extension of the patient.' In exploring this in more depth, nurses were seen to integrate the equip-ment into the total management of the patient. As such it became part of the assessment, intervention and evaluation process. It was an intrinsic part of the environment required to care for the patient.

In the intensive care environment, patient safety was a paramount issue in the use of the equipment. This led to standardised practice, in all of the units, of the nurse checking the equipment once patient handover at the bedside had been taken. This checking process was integrated as part of the patient assessment process and, on some units, required documentation on the observation chart. This practice has been described in other work (Scholes 1998). This process of getting organised was crucial to frame the patient in the environment and the results of this process were then used to inform subsequent decision making and interventions. As described in one field note entry:

> The nurse finished taking handover and then proceeded to introduce herself to the patient, although the patient was sedated and did not respond. She then moved behind the bed and checked equipment that could be required in an emergency, the suction, the oxygen. The patient was then assessed. This was undertaken systematically . . . respiratory, cardiovascular, renal. During this process, the relevant equipment was also checked; the ventilator was checked as part of the respiratory, the feeding pump as part of the nutrition or gastrointestinal assessment.

Nurses did not appear to acknowledge the technical information and practical skills required to co-ordinate this aspect of care and treatment into the multiplicity of needs of the critically ill. It was not identified as a source of credible knowledge. Yet this information was pertinent to clinical decision making. The equipment was a resource on the unit and nurses used this knowledge to ensure that care and treatment of the patient was timely and accurate. This resulted in nurses identifying the limitations of clinical decisions if there was a lack of resources: 'We'll need another line in if you want to start those antibiotics' or on another occasion: 'You'll have to stagger the filtration cycles as we only have three machines for the four patients.'

The nurses, as a result of their permanency in the units, demonstrated a high level of knowledge about the clinical environment and its resources. This informed the decisions made. In one ward round there was discussion about the fact that two patients needed a percutaneous tracheostomy performed on the unit that day:

> As the round concludes, there starts to develop banter about a race as to who can compete the task faster – the senior registrar or the medical consultant. This continues until the sister on for the unit adds: 'Yes, well you'll just have to wait until two sets of kit [sets of equipment] are available first.' The consultant says: 'Err, yes well that's a very good point.'

There are few nursing or sociological studies that identify nursing's use and co-ordination of equipment and of the health care environment. Indeed the nursing literature available is mainly critical of this knowledge. With a high focus on the use of technology in intensive care, this is seen to run counter to a person-centred philosophy of care. There is then inference that this works against the achievement of a holistic nurse–patient relationship (Fairman 1992). Conversely as argued by Pickles (1999), it here appeared that technology was being used to optimise the care delivered. Skilled and experienced nurses were able to work with the technology whilst remaining focused on the patient. However, these skills related to the equipment and appeared superfluous and unrecognised in the clinical decision making process.

There were many examples of nursing knowledge of the environment being used in decision making. As a relatively stable part of the workforce, nurses held a large knowledge store about the intensive care unit and the hospital. The nurses in charge were more familiar with the unit than most of the medical team, and therefore of its day-to-day working. This excerpt is from a conversation between a doctor to the nurse in charge:

> Doctor: Can we take two patients? Nurse: We'll discharge Mr W in bed 14 and Mr D in bed 2 to cardiac HDU and we can take two pumps. Doctor: Do we have Mr W – I didn't know we had him (laughs). Nurse: Yes he's the re-do CABG x 2. Extubated yesterday evening. No support.

Doing fine. Doctor: Oh, alright. So how many beds can we declare to EBS [emergency bed service]? Nurse: If we get Mrs C out today, then we have 1.

Nurses had developed a large repertoire of skills and knowledge in clinical unit management. Nurse managers were required to co-ordinate, manage, implement and troubleshoot. This required a working knowledge of the stores, supplies, personnel, and health and safety issues. It was through the work of the nursing team that the organisation of hospital policies such as the major incident procedures were locally agreed and implemented. This required substantial planning to cascade such information down to over a hundred staff in the largest of the units.

There were areas across the sites where projects had been delegated to the senior nurses by the manager or the clinical director. This expanded portfolio of nursing responsibilities has been well critiqued (Halford *et al.* 1997) and has required the development of its own unique knowledge base. Examples of such projects related to quality initiatives, and areas of stock, pharmacy and equipment administration. These were areas perceived by medicine and general managers to be: *nursing issues and to be dealt with by nurses.* Yet in reality nurses had little control over the use of resources in such areas. Although the responsibility to supervise these areas was placed on nurses, there was no authority to manage the resultant problems. For example, medical staff prescribed drugs, a costly unit expenditure over which nurses had no authority. If cost savings were required, this left nursing staff making suggestions on smaller and, at times, less consequential areas, such as dressings.

Nurses identified that resolution of problems in these areas therefore required debate, negotiation and creative thought. In this way they were termed by one nurse manager as 'non-decision areas'; those areas to which there was not an immediate solution: 'Non-decision things take time, those things that need to be done because there is no money. These are the things that are delegated out [to nurses].' This situation continues to reveal the inherent tension for nurses working concomitantly within Fordist and post-Fordist styles of management and working practices in the NHS as described by Walby and Greenwall (1994) nearly a decade ago. Medical staff also are being asked to manage this same tension working between historical, rigid, specialised divisions of labour and the call for more flexible, decentralised devolution of decision making. The difference is that medicine has greater control over how that process is managed.

The need for creative problem solving has further expanded nursing's knowledge of how to work within the organisation, and keep the system going. This enabled nurses to deliver a service whilst attempting to meet the demands of the managers and doctors:

You need to play the game with the managers and doctors – to know what each of them wants. You don't do anything different, just differently. You need to be more proactive and think how to respond to the different personalities. I go to the trust DNS [Director of Nursing] more with problems – I can be more candid as he understands it – he understands the different agendas that managers have.

The invisibility of the knowledge required to fully manage the environment, at the bedside and in the wider unit setting, is not entirely new to the literature. Liashensko (1998) explored how such knowledge, held by nurses, achieves a 'taken for granted' status within the organisational power structures. What is intriguing is how the more powerful discourses of medical and management operate to prevent recognition of this area of nursing knowledge that is central to the very functioning of the care delivery in the organisation.

Concluding thoughts

In this chapter, the domains of knowledge that are owned and used by nursing and medicine in decision making have been explored. The existence of a hierarchy of knowledge within patient and service management has been demonstrated. Within this, some critical issues have been highlighted that are pivotal to the understanding of the clinical decision-making process. Nurses and doctors in intensive care use both shared and discrete types of knowledge. Even in intensive care, an area where nurses can articulate a strong clinical and management knowledge base within their own areas of practice, the medical worldview of knowledge remains dominant in making decisions in health care.

Medical and managerial staff are not uninformed of the knowledge that nurses possess. Doctors and managers can identify specific area of expertise underpinned by nursing knowledge. Nonetheless, the decision-making agenda and forum structures do not accommodate nursing issues *per se* and an interdisciplinary forum to truly demonstrate nursing knowledge and expertise is lacking. Despite the depth and extent of nursing knowledge, it is not well used and has little impact on decision making in intensive care. Because of this, nursing knowledge is not valued in either clinical or management practice and the traditional medical and managerial hegemony are sustained.

Chapter 7

Roles in clinical decision making

Working with a historical legacy

An important issue to emerge from consideration of decision making in the clinical setting was the nature of medical and nursing roles. This included how doctors and nurses described their roles in the decision-making process, and how doctors and nurses demonstrated these roles in the clinical environment. In this chapter, both these elements are described and explored further through reference to work undertaken on the division of labour.

At its most basic level, examination of the decision-making process between doctors and nurses in intensive care revealed a recurrent pattern that demonstrated the respective roles adopted. The following field note excerpt demonstrates this:

> Nurse [to doctor]: 'Come and look at this drain. It's making a hideous noise and causing a huge air leak.' The nurse takes down the dressing and prepares the site for the doctor, then gets pad and new dressing. The doctor looks at the drain: 'I can put a stitch in it if you want, it doesn't really matter . . . The nurse finally says: 'Well OK, put one in then.' The doctor renews the stitch and then as he leaves the room: 'I'll leave you to dress it.'

This incident simplistically distinguishes the different role functions identified in clinical decision making. In explicating this at its most fundamental level, the nurse in surveying the patient as part of nursing work, identified a problem (increased air leak). Through the nurse highlighting this issue to the doctor, the decision-making process was then informed. From this, a decision was made (to place a suture), and this was then implemented (new suture inserted). Throughout this, the environment was managed to enable the process of care to continue (area prepared for procedure, and wound re-dressed afterwards).

Through analysis of these events, key issues are now explored concerning: how nurses survey their working environment; the nature of authority within the decision-making process; how the decisions that are made are then worked with; and the need to manage the environment in which decision making is undertaken.

Surveillance work

It was clear that much of the work of both doctors and nurses within the intensive care was related to surveillance. I am using the word 'surveillance' simply to describe a monitoring role and work undertaken as part of the process of making clinical decisions, not with a specific sociological orientation that others have used (Foucault 1975). As detailed in the previous chapter, the framework employed to inform clinical decisions used data collected from the close monitoring of the patient. Much of the therapy in intensive care was not directly curative, but supportive. In this way, mechanical ventilation was used to support the patient's breathing until the primary problem had resolved. This then required monitoring to ensure that adequate supportive therapy was being given. Therefore routine observations and tests were carried out to direct optimal therapy. The nurse, being at the bedside, was in a prime position to monitor and survey the patient in this way.

As a result of this principal nursing surveillance role, there was a reliance on the nurse to identify and communicate immediate problems. If the blood pressure fell, for example, the nurse noted this and reported it to the medical staff. In this fashion, problems were highlighted that required resolution. More experienced nurses had developed an expanded surveillance role in which they not only surveyed parameters considered to be an essential part of nursing observations (for example, heart rate and rhythm, ventilator observations), but also included monitoring of drug levels, blood results and necessary intravenous lines changes. The results of such observations were documented on the observation chart or in the patient's notes. As discussed in Chapter 6, it was often such surveillance information that medical staff used to inform patient presentation on formal ward rounds. This information was used even if it had been a busy shift when the doctor on call may not have seen the patient. In this situation, there was usually a brief handover from the nurse to the doctor, giving relevant medical details for the doctor to then present on the round. This is demonstrated in the following extract:

> Doctor [to nurse]: So anything happened overnight? Nurse: Weaned the ventilation, she's now on 50 per cent and pressure support of 14. Inotropes off, good pressures. Spiked a pyrexia, still on her antibiotics. Good urine output. Coming down on the sedation and she's settled.

This situation was a 'taken for granted practice' in all units. Nurses supplied the specific patient information, which was then channelled through medicine. Neither medical nor nursing staff acknowledged that it was predominantly nursing work that was at times used *verbatim* in the medical handover that was then used directly to inform patient decisions.

As discussed previously, it was the medical framework that was utilised for presentation on the ward round. It was often presumed by medical staff that nurses were there to raise issues that may have been overlooked by the medical team: 'I would therefore expect the experienced nurse to chip in, to alert me to things that we've missed out.' These issues had either been omitted from the original presentation within the medical framework, or lay outside of this framework. Nurses were therefore placed in a role to collate patient information and bring this to the attention of the medical staff who then acted on it.

In perceiving such functions as part of the technical division of labour (Hughes 1984), nurses collected and monitored patient data, and medical staff presented these as part of patient assessment in the decision-making forums. These were the socially agreed boundaries that were used to describe roles within decision making. However, as asserted by Hughes (*op. cit.*), empirical work should focus on what people actually do, and not what they think they do. In describing what both medical and nursing staff actually do, the nursing skills required to bring together patient information; the decisions taken on what information to raise and not raise; and the decisions made by nursing staff during the surveillance process were disregarded by medical and nursing staff alike.

The growing complexity of intensive care has increased the intricacy of patient surveillance. If an occupation is a bundle of tasks (Hughes *op. cit.*), by mapping the tasks that nurses have had to perform in the past, the historical development of the nursing role can be recognised. Despite nurses performing more complicated tasks requiring more detailed knowledge and skills to carry out, the function of nursing surveillance is not perceived as a valued activity within the division of labour.

On the ward round, nurses did not routinely present details of specific nursing issues for the patient. Therefore events such as moving the patient onto a different bed, complex wound dressings, or activities requiring some organisation including sitting the patient out of bed, or hair washing was not reported on by nurses. Instead, nurses were often silent in the ward round. Their role was mainly confined to supplying further detail of the patient if required by medical staff:

> As the junior anaesthetist is presenting the patient, the consultant is examining the chart and then the patient. If anything needs clarifying or if a specific update on events is required – he looks around and says – Where's nursey?

In this way, nursing continued to be defined in terms of its usefulness to medicine and management in health care, and not through its primary contribution to the patient's and the service management. Nursing continued to be defined principally in terms of instrumental medical functions (Alaszewski 1995). In undertaking these technical competencies, nurses continued to function as unseen, highly skilled workers (Lawler 1997).

Further details were often sought from nurses if the medical information was not current. This occurred if units were busy. Medical staff had to oversee the progress of all patients, where nurses mainly looked after one patient for the duration of that shift. As reflected in this excerpt about one patient's ventilatory management, patient treatments can quickly change:

> Junior doctor presenting on the round: Well, we've kept her sedated and fully ventilated overnight. Consultant asks nurse: How's she doing now? Nurse replies: We've weaned her onto support mode and she's coping well.

During such times, nurses often adopted a more proactive approach in the ward round and, in the absence of medical knowledge of the patient, the nurse led the patient presentation. As one consultant highlighted: 'Nurses are there to confirm and point out what was important, especially if sometimes the doctor has been in bed all night.' On larger, busier units or those with less medical cover, the doctors had little time to become acquainted with some of the patients. This led to nurses having a role beyond the traditional surveillance role. On one unit, the consultants acknowledged that this situation challenged historical perceptions of the nursing role: 'The unit is large. We're lucky to have, without exception very good G grades. They have a high level of knowledge in ICU and more experience than all the SHOs together. Especially during the nights, they make the decisions.'

This raises an interesting issue. It appeared to me that the nursing role on this unit was identical to the other sites in this study. However here, the nurses had frequent opportunity of reporting directly on the ward round what patient problems had occurred, and how these had been managed. It was through this opportunity for nurses to present their actual surveillance work, rather than have doctors report on this, that affirmed what the nurses undertook on the unit. This gave nurses the public voice to demonstrate the nature and value of their work.

There was a resonance in how information was collected and used by all the health care team in developing in service management. Again, it was the nurses and non-medical staff who mainly gathered data that was used for problem solving. Just as clinical information was obtained through the continuous monitoring of the patients, there were similar parallel examples within the service development forums. Service decision-making issues were informed by data that was collected by ward clerks, audit staff, nurses and, to some degree, by managers. Areas that were surveyed included stores, staffing, patient throughput, bed occupancy and audit. This was then used in service decision making.

In observing the activity of the nursing staff, it was clear that data collection comprised a substantial part of their role, but nursing did not have control over what data was collected. Whenever new equipment was introduced, new hospital procedures initiated, or another medical research study carried out on the unit, it was the nursing staff who were required to add further observations or charting to their surveillance role. Again, nurses were carrying out medical and managerial work with little acknowledgement. It was concerning that this was not recognised by doctors; but it was more concerning that it was not recognised by nurses either.

Recognised authority and unrecognised responsibility

A key issue within decision making was who carried the authority and the responsibility of making clinical decisions. The vast majority of formal clinical decisions were made by doctors, or in the service decision-making development, by doctors and managers. This fact was not only observable but also emerged from the interviews, and was revealed in the documentation. One doctor asserted that:

> Medical staff have the responsibility to make the decisions and lead the process of care. To set the plan for the day or for the week. To set the priorities of care and evaluate the treatment plan. They are to take note of the input from the sources but he is responsible and he must make the decisions. One can't be too forbidding, *but I must maintain control – that's what I'm paid for.*

Doctors identified that they held power in decision making through the knowledge and position they held in the organisation; this was reflected in the salary that doctors commanded. Medical power results from medicine's ability to diagnose and treat illness (Jolley and Brykczyskia 1993) and this leads to medical dominance in decision making. Nurses work within the decisions that are made, and therefore function in a supportive role (Walby and Greenwall 1994). Once again, the status of nursing is derived from the norms of medical behaviour and technical cure (Jones 1987).

This primary role function by medicine was recognised by, and was perceived to arise from, the medical staffs' professional responsibilities and role remit. Doctors equally held strong views about the position adopted by nursing during the decision-making process: '*But I take the can. Nurses won't take that decision. They won't say, but they want their input.* After all I feel I have the knowledge and I'm being paid to make those decisions.' The opinion being expressed was categorically clear. Doctors identified that nurses were aspiring to have input into decisions, but that nurses did not put their view forward, nor take the responsibility that came with it. Perhaps such opinions put forward by doctors can be best illustrated in the following, not uncommon example. The event during which these notes were made occurred during a post-operative patient review by a surgeon: 'No eye contact with nurse or patient. Doesn't ask any questions of the nurse. Nurse doesn't volunteer any information. Doctor uses his finger along the chart: Yes, yes, yes . . . Keep the dopamine on. OK all going well. He turns and leaves.' Within both clinical and service decision-making arenas, the medical role in making the decisions was explicit, the nursing role was subservient and, at times, passive.

There were, however, clear examples of a consultative working environment during the ward round. This occurred especially if difficult decisions were being made: 'Doctor: So we've decided to pull out, is everyone happy with that? Pause – all nod. Doctor: Right, I'll see the family.' There were also other times when there was dissent expressed by nurses about the decisions made. Such concerns were not always presented at the time of the ward round, but more frequently expressed afterwards in company with other nursing staff. After a ward round discussion regarding the management of a long-term sick patient, one nurse was obviously frustrated: *It's easy for them, they can just turn their back and leave the room*. The doctors have endoscoped the patient and it's NAD [nothing abnormal detected]. *But they just won't do anything.* They don't realise the aspiration sets patients back 4–5 days weaning. I just wish they'd stop trying to feed her and put a TPN [total parenteral nutrition] line in and leave it until she's off the vent. Such conversations often occurred away from the immediate clinical work, for example in the coffee room. The question here is: why nurses did not feel that they could raise their concerns on the round? Nurses often complained that they felt that the doctors would not listen to their views, or that they felt intimidated when challenging doctors on the ward round. In such situations, nurses remained silent on the round, leaving the nurses unhappy with the decisions being made. This later led to tension and conflict of which the medical staff were unaware.

Although it was generally held that doctors made most of the decisions in intensive care, it was not an automatic assumption that nurses made no decisions. One consultant acknowledged:

> Nurses make judgements that the patient is stable and when to be turned etc. – the minute by minute decisions. Medical decisions are related to the type of treatment, the tests ordered etc. There is clearly a huge overlap between who is responsible for what. Doctors set the parameters and nurses can work within those parameters.

Despite the above assertion, the fact that nurses did exercise decision making within patient management was generally poorly recognised by either nurses or doctors. When observing in the field, there were many examples of nurses making decisions. Experienced nurses would often take the initiative and start to reduce the drugs and oxygen being given if the patient was becoming more stable. One nurse was talking through her plan: 'Well, he's got good pressures [blood pressure] so I'm going to start weaning off the adren [adrenaline]. He doesn't need it any more.' These actions were then reported on the ward round as fact.

Decision making by nurses did not just occur within the clinical domain. There were similar examples of nurses making decisions within the service decision-making arena: 'The manager is quite supportive . . . The day-to-day management is left up to us. We need authorisation about staffing – but we hardly ever see managers.' Although managers did influence some aspects of unit decision making, nurses managed other areas entirely independently. Even with such acknowledged blurring of the role boundaries between nursing, medicine and management with regards to decision making, it was generally agreed that decision making was a medical and managerial activity. In not acknowledging the increasing unrecognised authority and responsibility that nurses held in these areas, nursing's dependence on medicine and management was reinforced.

In the current situation of dynamic working and organic boundaries between medicine and nursing, there is a challenge to the historical presumption about care and cure, in which it is deemed that only doctors can diagnose and pre-scribe. In the sociological literature, such border lines are seen to be historically and socially, rather than functionally defined (Walby and Greenwall 1994). Medicine and nursing are seen as part of a larger, and not necessarily distinct division of labour. It is the control of the division of labour by medicine that is distinct (Freidson 1970). In the field, local necessity and demand was requiring medicine to allow traditional divisions of labour to flex, although this continued to remain firmly under medicine's control.

Medicine's jurisdiction over traditional role boundaries was clearly evident. Certain clinical decisions required a specific medical authority before nursing action could be undertaken. On one unit, one nurse remarked: 'I'd take bloods, and take the results to the docs and ask then if I can extubate. They usually tell us what we know in any case, but it needs a doctor's OK.' Even if knowledge was held as to the correct course of action, sanction had to be sought from the person holding the authority to make that decision. The impetus for seeking medical sanction was more evident if the required action fell outside the inter-pretation generally held in that unit, of what the boundaries of the nursing role were. Again, this was contextually bound: the procedures or decisions nurses undertook on one unit, may not have been undertaken on the other sites. This created frustration as nurses moved from one unit to another. The need for nurses to seek medical authority for something they had previously been able to carry out independently elsewhere appeared unnecessary, was not seen to acknowledge individual skills, and was felt to prolong treatment times for patients.

In Durkheim's (1933) work on sexual division of labour, it can be seen how, historically, health care work has been compatibly divided between nurses and doctors. Traditionally, nursing has been largely a female profession, and medi-cine, a male profession. This gendered system of health care succeeded because medical and nursing work followed different objectives, directed by the need to cure or care. Contemporary health care has dramatically changed. Medical and nursing roles no longer have discrete functions. There are now areas of shared knowledge and to some extent, shared functions. As has been demon-strated in this chapter, this inevitably leads to friction and tension between doctors and nurses.

Working with decisions

Once clinical decisions were made, this became the plan for clinical and service practice. All groups worked with the decisions made, clinical staff implementing clinical decision making, managers and clinical staff implementing service decision making. However, it was nurses whose primary role was to implement and work the decisions that were made across the clinical and service domains. In the clinical arena, once the patient had been seen during the ward round, the nurse was then left to continue care and treatment. Following the decisions made on the ward round, nurses made fine manipulations of the patient treatment whilst working within the parameters set. To some extent, nurses across all the units altered patient ventilation, sedation, and inotropes as required, and managed intravenous fluids, feeding and haemofiltration. There were similarities within the service area. Once budget levels had been set, nurses acted to ensure that such areas were managed to meet the target set. If local trust policy was cascaded down to units, nursing staff acted to ensure implementation was successful. The local planning of such projects was within the domain of the senior nursing team.

This gave rise to some interesting issues. There were some practice areas where, after an initial covering order had been given by medical staff, nurses were able to make their own clinical decisions. In the clinical arena, this was most notable in the administration of certain drugs and fluids. Often a standard list was written up, and so nurses could instigate sedation and administer fluids at their own discretion. The legality of some of these prescriptions was debatable. In extremely sick patients, these prescriptions often acted as a guide. The amount of drug required by the patient often exceeded the amount originally prescribed, thereby rendering the prescription obsolete. New junior medical staff on the units often asked nurses what drug was preferred in that unit, and how to prescribe it. In responding to these questions, the nurse was performing supplementary prescribing, in all but writing the prescription. Such observations are not new (Walby and Greenwall 1994) but within the current study, these were further examples of the unrecognised and unofficial decision making undertaken by intensive care nurses in working with patient managements.

Despite prevailing historical practices and attitudes, there was evidence that traditional perceptions of role function were changing. Across all sites there was a general recognition that role boundaries were shifting. Within this, nurses were seen to be taking on more clinically developed roles. This was seen by doctors to include the support of junior medical staff: 'I think we need to realise that really the E grade staff nurses are experienced in intensive care and it is them who actually instruct the junior medical staff. I mean really now nurses are doing everything except actually writing up the drugs.'

Such role changes placed nurses in a position to make decisions and influence the management of decisions about patients. As one doctor remarked:

The nurse's job description has changed and the doctors on ICU are getting younger. Consultants in the days of the extended role saw this as a barrier to learning. In ICU, this is really the 'normal role', part of their everyday job, not an extended role. The attitude to nurses by medicine has changed. 10 years ago, medicine would *never* have worked with a pain management sister.

It was evident that nursing roles have dramatically altered in contemporary health care. Although nursing initially established its credibility through nurses' proficient implementation of doctors' orders, the nursing role has since evolved to include a more critical understanding, interpretation and application of these instructions. This aspect of the nursing role was not well acknowledged by doctors and nurses in the interviews, and yet was clearly evident from observations in the field. Nurses working with the decision parameters ensured that patients received timely interventions. This is demonstrated in the discussion with a nurse about the extubation of her patient:

> He's got good gases, on minimal support, good lung expansion, no pain and he wants the tube out. The doctor wants to wait until the ward round, but the patient wants the tube out and I think we only have a small window for this man's successful extubation given his previous history.

Nurses working with such decisions had potential benefit for patients, ensured that resources were utilised effectively, and helped to ensure that neither medicine nor the system became overloaded. Whilst nurses working in this way was not recognised by doctors or nurses, it was immediately noted when it became absent from normal working practices and roles. This situation could be precipitated by a very junior member of the nursing staff caring for a patient, or by a nurse who was not prepared to flex traditional working boundaries. As highlighted by one consultant: 'Like the other day, I made a flippant throw away comment about a head injury that was going to die – I made a throw away comment about "We'll have to watch the K [potassium]." The next thing I know was that the nurse had urgently bleeped the doctor saying "the K's rising".' The inexperienced nurse had literally interpreted the consultant's remark and therefore made, in the consultant's opinion, an unnecessary urgent bleep. It appeared that the nurse's role in this area was almost invisible to those involved in clinical decision making until, it was removed.

The difference between having authority to make decisions and the responsibility to work with the decisions previously made was a key issue for medical and nursing staff on the units. All consultants stated that they had overall authority and accountability for the unit, and left the nursing staff responsible to manage the clinical care and service. Nurses equally held this view. One senior nurse spoke about her role:

> I am responsible for the quality and audit . . . of auditing the nursing function and meeting the trust requirements for standard setting and audit.

I have to cover risk management and critical incident reporting. I work with the clinical director on clinical audit . . . the majority of this work is undertaken or led by nurses [she smirks].

In reality, this meant that the power to make decisions rested with the medical staff and the managers. Nurses were responsible for implementing and working with the decisions that were made and over which they had minimal influence or control. The nursing influence was confined to how those decisions were implemented and managed.

Medical and nursing staff had different perceptions on the impact of management on the decision-making process. All the senior nurses identified the need to build effective working relationships with managers, but some medical staff adopted a more radical view:

Regards my relationship with management – well they don't impact really. I really only get concerned if they detract my available resources. I adopt a position of detached disinterest. I just keep them occupied and away from us. There is very few obstacles placed by management – *we are very much on top of them . . . All of us are pugnacious little bastards.* We have a very tame clinical director and the speciality manager has not tried to take us on – we are a tightly run unit.

In all the sites, this had the effect of creating a hierarchy within the service decision-making domain. Medical staff, assisted by the fact that the clinical director was a consultant, had the authority to make decisions within the clinical and service arena. Managers also had the power base to direct service decision making but mainly by their direct authority over the nursing staff. This resulted in a consensus view that the nursing role in decision making was confined to informing the decision-making process, and working with the decisions. The nursing authority over the total decision-making process was limited. As highlighted in a study by Cott (1997), 'I decide, you carry it out' had simply become 'We decide, you carry it out.'

The organisational glue

There were incidents in the field that pointed to the importance of managing the clinical and service environment to enable the decision-making process to proceed smoothly. It was difficult to determine whether these roles had been formally designated to specific groups or adopted by those groups as no one else was undertaking them. Managing the environment was demonstrated not through centre stage decisions made about patients admitted into the units, but about setting up and resourcing bed space for that patient. It was not about making decisions to open an extra intensive care bed, but about how and when that bed was going to be opened. It was the nurse who most frequently managed the environment in this way and acted as the organisational glue that enabled the clinical and service domains to function.

This nursing role was most obvious at the bedside during the ward round. During this time, it was predominantly the nurses who drew the curtains round the patient, explain to the patient what was happening, make the patient comfortable and return any equipment. In this way, the ward round could proceed smoothly with maximum preparation and minimal interruption.

As previously described, this became part of the nurses' role to manage the patient's bed space during their shift. Such environmental work did not appear to be part of the doctor's role as this extreme example demonstrates: 'Doctor comes to examine patient – leaves stethoscope on the bed, goes to the patient, completely examines the patient without saying anything, doctor walks away. Nurse starts to tidy sheets and bed area.' Through the checking and ordering of equipment around the bed, this space became territory over which the nurse presided. As a general observation, imposition by other staff within this space appeared to occur with little challenge.

As nurses were the constant element of the workforce, they also monitored wider clinical management issues. All of the units had set protocols, for example, changing of intravenous lines or, for long-term patient, setting up case conferences. It was the nursing staff who had the responsibility to manage this aspect of clinical environment for the patient. In talking about case conferences, one nurse remarks: 'It is still up to us to let the consultants know when the 28 days are up.' This concept of overseeing the environment also extended to general unit issues. The following situation occurred at the end of the ward round:

> After this the anaesthetist then pointed to the water on the floor and suggested that 'she could perhaps mop it up' as it could be a potential electrical hazard with the electrical cable nearby. The round then left. I could see that the nurse was upset by these events so I went back to talk to her. She was livid. 'I've never felt so embarrassed . . . and when the anaesthetist pointed out the electrical cable and the water on the floor, I felt so humiliated. Was that all they could say? And then to turn as an afterthought and ask if there was anything – I've never been so embarrassed.'

Equally, the nurse managers worked to ensure that all resources were available to achieve the overall smooth running of the unit. Key important areas identified by nursing staff included ordering of staff, disposable equipment, and other resources required to maintain the unit's functioning. Management of this area was seen as an implicit part of the senior nursing role, and was formally recognised in all senior nursing job descriptions. It was the senior nurses who, using their knowledge of the unit and of the patients on the unit, ensured that any resources required to deliver the service plan be available. This included negotiating with pharmacy, sterile supplies, other clinical areas, and agencies for nursing staff to cover shifts. Such day-to-day issues were not on the agendas of the key decision-making forums, and yet were crucial to enable the unit to deliver the commissioned service. These areas were only located onto the formal agendas if financial or service delivery problems were encountered.

This situation presents a real dichotomy. The nursing role was perceived by medical staff and managers to be subservient in terms of decision making, and yet essential to ensure that the necessary decisions were made and put into practice. Nurses were required by medical staff to adopt an institutional role of self-disciplined servants to prepare and make good the environment, but equally be professionally educated to intelligently apply and evaluate decisions made. Nurses are therefore simultaneously being asked to be a flexible workforce of professionally motivated carers, and required to complete tasks that are not owned by others (Chapman 1976). For nurses this creates a paradox of roles: to be marginal to medicine in decision making, and yet central to medicine in the delivery of health care practice.

Nurses function as the 'intermediary between the doctor and the patient . . . and simultaneously as the interface between the patient and the potentially bureaucratic nature of the health service' Mackay (1989, p. 4). Nurses routinely undertake informal, unrecognised practices required to sustain organisational work (Jolley and Brykcznski 1993). Such taken-for-granted activities in roles have already received attention in the nursing (Davies 1995; Cohen 1995), secretarial (Pringle 1989), and clerical health service (Saks 1990) literature. A feminist reading of this area acknowledges women as undertaking facilitating work within an organisation holding implicit masculine approaches to problem solving and interaction (Gilligan 1982). Gamarnikow (1991) believes that both doctors and nurses accept the subordinate position of nursing in the division of labour. Medicine dominates – justified on grounds of female obedience – whilst nurses perceive the subordination to be based on the functional nature of their respective roles.

Nurses as an occupational group are predominantly practice based, and female. Abbott (1988) argues that an occupational structure is historically segregated by gender. This has traditionally led to women's position within their public role as being taken from their role in private: of having a primary responsibility for managing the home. Nursing is fundamentally perceived as women's work, and therefore undervalued (Gamarnikow 1991; Witz 1992). Nursing roles in decision making may therefore be perceived as nurses undertaking decision-making 'housework' for doctors and managers. Doctors make key decisions, and nurses prepare, work with, and highlight any problems in decision making.

Nurses continue to take on an increased number of tasks and responsibilities from doctors and managers as indicated by the changing role of the nurse in intensive care (RCN 1997). As discussed, this change has not been balanced with an increased level of authority (Annandale 1996), further re-affirming nursing's subordination to medicine (Hugman 1991).

Concluding thoughts

It is clear that within the decision-making process, medicine continues to maintain its superiority. Despite nursing and management role developments, the historical legacy of medical dominance in decision making is maintained. This is achieved through medicine's explicit authority to make decisions and the continued importance placed on the function of making decisions. The impact of such dominance is that the significance of other roles required to inform, implement and manage the decisions made is neglected. In an era of increased focus on governance and interdisciplinary working, this reinforces the need for all to value team contributions to patient and service management.

In this chapter, I have demonstrated that the nursing role in the decision-making process is more varied and multi-faceted than previously thought. Nurses utilise diverse knowledge sources to inform the decision-making process through their surveillance work, then work with the decision, and support the environment to enable the decisions to be implemented. It is clear that the contribution of nursing to the decision-making process cannot be judged by the degree of authority that nursing holds to make decisions; the very role function that both nursing and medicine continue to hold in high regard. What is obvious is that neither nurses, medicine nor managers value the wider roles that nursing contributes to the decision-making process.

This chapter has both reinforced and challenged the rhetoric of functional nursing roles. Nursing is inherently an ambiguous activity, a boundary discipline, sitting on a dynamic decision-making stage. Traditional role boundaries and concepts are constantly questioned. As described by Freidson (1976), the division of labour is defined and re-defined by the social interaction of medicine and nursing, within the existing constraints. It is the existence of the constraints that is the key issue. At all the study sites, there was some evidence of change in the division of labour in order to deliver contemporary health care. Such changes are occurring in individual units and remain only locally acknowledged. As a result, such role re-definitions are not universally acknowledged and remain otherwise invisible. Therefore, the power and authority that rests with specific roles and professional groups are not substantially changing.

Nurses are seen to have an important role in the intensive care unit (Jowett 1986) and the primary care led NHS (Caines 1996). Both medical and nursing staff bring a range of roles and skills to the decision-making process. However, descriptions of nursing and medical roles remain attributed to the disciplines with which they have been traditionally associated. A focus on the organisational and contextual issues may transcend the orthodox model of professionalism in order to effect change (Salvage 1988) and thereby enable new partnerships and participation between doctors and nurses to emerge (Davies 1995).

Chapter 8

Power and conflict on the clinical decision-making stage

This chapter explores the themes of power and conflict between doctors and nurses in decision making in intensive care. In this study, medical and nursing staff described themselves as working as part of cohesive clinical team, and this indeed was demonstrated the majority of the time. However, in the decision-making process, nursing perceived medicine to be domineering, and medicine perceived nursing to be weak, wanting a voice, but unprepared to take the concomitant responsibility. The power of each discipline and the conflict between them were made manifest through the knowledge used for, and the roles used in, decision making. The way in which this happened is explored together with the strategies used by both medicine and nursing to manage the resultant conflict.

In order to explore and analyse this phenomenon further, I have used a range of literature but have particularly chosen to use a dramaturgical perspective (Goffman 1959). In this chapter, I explain the rationale for this particular lens to focus on the decision-making stage, and then apply this theatrical metaphor to provide a further theoretical perspective on the decision-making process and the nursing role in this area of practice.

Setting the stage

The process of decision making in intensive care could have represented an integrated way of working with nurses and doctors holding complementary knowledge bases and roles. Indeed, there were examples of mutually satisfying, well-developed relationships between medicine and nurses: 'There appears to be a very open relationship between the consultant and the nursing staff. Nurse: What time are you doing the ward round? Consultant: Three minutes. Nurse looks thoughtful. Consultant: Ten minutes OK then? Nurse: Yes that's fine.' Flexible working arrangements were demonstrated, and all participants were optimistic about the general working relationships between medicine and nursing.

Nurses and doctors spoke positively about working relationships in intensive care. However, within the specific area of decision making, the working relationships were not perceived by nursing or medicine to be so mutual or satisfying. All participants held strong opinions about this area. This is clearly demonstrated in the following extract where the senior nurse is describing the nursing role on the unit:

> the nursing staff have expanded their role tremendously since then and have very much been allowed to develop within reason . . . It is truly a reflection of our relationship with the medical staff. They [the nurses] are truly accountable for their actions and their planning of care; they really look at what they are going to achieve, and how they are going to achieve it.

This extract reflects a very positive account of team working. However, only minutes earlier in the interview, the senior nurse had been describing the response of the nursing team to the behaviour of one consultant during the ward round: 'They are threatened or intimidated by his manner and that is where we need to be supporting our nursing staff.' As a result of such behaviour, the team dynamics were affected, resulting in nurses feeling unable to contribute to the decision-making process. This gave rise to conflict in decision making in that clinical setting.

An enduring theme across the data concerned how decisions were made in intensive care, and who had input into that process. Whilst these points were raised by all study participants, nursing and medicine had different interpretations on this:

> Nurse: I would like to see the ward rounds develop. I would like them to be shorter [laughs] and more democratic – to get more involved, especially given the increased amount of responsibility on nurses at present. *I would like greater control over the process*, over the way it is discussed.

Nurses were persistent in their belief that decision making was controlled by medicine, leaving little opportunity for influence by nurses. This was contrasted with a strong belief from doctors about medical power in decision making:

> *Nursing is very rigid* – they are always showing fear, always covering their back. Medicine is a profession – nursing isn't. Medicine and law are professions: no regulations, self-governing, experienced experts in their field. *No one will seek to constrain us with rules* and regulations. Guidelines – *well they're a load of bollocks*. Nurses are highly skilled but have always been regulated. They are expected to comply with rules, they develop procedures. Medicine doesn't, we are free agents. Medicine tries controversial procedures, my nurses are constrained within a framework – which are produced in vast arrays of paperwork which really doesn't have a great deal of relevance to clinical practice.

Doctors did not perceive themselves to be part of the structure that constrained nursing and did therefore not reflect on the possibility that the medical role placed restrictions on nursing. Medical staff did not acknowledge how they themselves reinforced the rigid framework within which nurses found themselves, nor how they influenced the use of nursing knowledge and nursing roles within patient and service management arenas.

There were many decision-making situations that revealed the use of power and conflict arising from tensions such as those described. However, there was one particular incident, which for me contained all these elements. It concerned a discussion on the use of an invasive monitoring tool, colloquially known as a Swan Ganz catheter. This ward round situation is presented in full, to act as an introduction to this section.

> The senior registrar puts forward a suggestion for a CT scan for a patient who has become increasingly unstable and unresponsive to treatments overnight. The consultant asks what information the scan will give and the senior registrar gives a brief rationale about detail on the patient's lung function and diagnoses. The consultant replies: A bit on the edge there, we'll hold that one. The patient had continued to require a lot of volume [blood and intravenous fluids], and yet the blood pressure was continuing to sag. The nurse in charge then asks consultant if inserting a Swan Ganz catheter would help. The consultant turns to the nurse and says: '*Why? So he can have a nice yellow thing sticking out of his neck [laughs] Why?*' The nurse answers: 'So that we can measure his cardiac function.' Now the rest of the round is silent, everyone is listening. The consultant replies: '*No it's just that he's sick and you think he needs a Swan. Tell me, why do you think he needs Swan?*' The nurse's face is reddening and you can start to hear her voice becoming nervous. She is starting to look at the patient rather than at the consultant. She answers: 'I just feel that he has needed increasing amounts of volume overnight, and we're not getting anywhere with his pressure.' The consultant replies: '*Well we'll put a Swan in if it makes you happy, yes, we'll put one in and that will tell us what we already know. That he's got a bad heart and we'll take it out and carry on treating him as we already are,* but yes we'll put one in if it makes you happy. It will cost the earth and put the patient at risk of further problems.' The nurse starts to protest: 'No it's just that . . .' She looks around for further support. The rest of the round remains quiet and no one makes any response. They move on to the next patient with no apparent concrete plan for the patient except 'just continue'. As they move away the nurse says to the other doctors: '*Thanks for your help back there.*' She is obviously irritated and upset by the event. The consultant by this time had gone to wash his hands, returns and starts in a more measured tone to discuss the Swan incident again. Before the next patient is presented, he turns with a smile on his face to the nurse in charge and says: 'I don't mind you suggesting and discussing things, it is important. But we need to

rationalise what we do and ensure they benefit the patient.' After the round had finished, several doctors joined me and started talking about this incident: 'You know he would have challenged us in exactly the same way. She was right, she just didn't push the point home. In any case, we agree with her, before long, he'll have a Swan in.'

I then recorded in my field notes that the 'Swan saga' continued. The patient unfortunately became increasingly unstable during the day, and by early evening a Swan Ganz catheter had been inserted. On the next ward round, the same nurse in charge comments to the same consultant: '"So, I see you had to put a Swan in then. *Tell me, why exactly did you put a Swan in?*" He replied: "Because I was told on the ward round to put one in [laughs]." The conversation is terminated.'

A key issue raised in this incident is conflict over the use of knowledge during review of the patient. The knowledge used by the consultant dominated over the rationale put forward by the nurse. Through knowledge, medicine was able to exert its power over nursing. Medicine had the ability to direct and use that knowledge through the principal role of directing decision making. Through power held in this role, any challenges to medical knowledge, or alternative decision-making actions were thereby dismissed. Power in this process was equally displayed through medicine not being required to justify the knowledge used, and by the derogatory manner in which the alternative suggestions were treated.

The actions of the junior medical staff who clearly agreed with the suggestion put forward by the nurse and yet did not challenge the consultant nor openly support the nurse, were also noted. The lack of support from junior doctors for nurses in decision-making forums was well recognised by nurses across the sites. Whatever the underlying basis was for this behaviour, it was interpreted by nursing staff as a lack of moral character in the doctors:

> I'm saddened by junior doctors of today, their lack of integrity is very disconcerting. Very few of them challenge the consultants. I may have been arguing or discussing that I don't agree. The consultant stands there and the senior registrar stands there, and I argue. And when the consultant leaves he says 'I agree with you.' So I ask why they didn't say so at the time – and I never get an answer. *And you call it a democratic process.*

Nurses felt that they had become a lone voice presenting an alternative view in decision making. This was a source of distress to nurses who perceived decision making as a democratic process, having the capacity to be informed and contributed to by any individual. As there was no other dissenting voice to medicine, nursing staff felt left to fight in isolation, requiring both emotional and moral courage.

Power and knowledge: the marginalisation of nursing

As has been discussed in earlier chapters, both nurses and doctors recognised that in order to effectively influence decision making, the use of rational, objective scientific or financial knowledge was required. Such knowledge was put forward to justify suggestions made, in order for these to be considered during the making of decisions:

> Some of the more junior [nursing] staff know what they want to say and have an idea of what they want to achieve, but have a hard time justifying it. And I think a lot of them realise that until they can justify what they want to do, they'll have a hard time getting accepted by the medical staff.

Although this situation was unconditionally accepted by medicine, nursing felt that subjective or wider nursing knowledge and issues were ignored. Nurses interpreted this as they themselves were being ignored. The following situation is illustrative of many incidents. I was talking to one nurse at the bedside. Two doctors were standing by the observation chart, pointing and talking. The nurse reflected: 'it makes you feel like a *second class citizen*, and when you speak they just think, oh, it's that *nursey* thing again.'

As previously explored, medical staff placed importance on the bedside nurse having intimate knowledge of the patient, although this knowledge was not frequently used as a source of information in decision making. When this source of nursing knowledge was overlooked, or not acknowledged, nurses felt frustrated and devalued. The following powerful incident concerns the management of a patient who, in the nurse's view, had become distressed. The nurse was asking the medical staff permission to administer further sedative drugs. After presenting her case, the consultant asks:

> 'What do you think her sedation score is right now?' Behind the nurse at other side of bed, the senior registrar is attempting to elicit a gag response by tugging at the ETT [endotracheal tube]. This action is noted by the round and all giggle. The nurse looks round. Consultant says: '−2, therefore the answer is no, wean the midazolam off.' Nurse: '*but she was agitated before, we've just given her sedation for physio*. [physiotherapy]'. Consultant: 'Well, we're doing a trachy soon, leave the midazolam off as it will defeat the object of the exercise in achieving a quick wean.' Nurse looks upset and angry and obviously unhappy with the exchange.

In this situation, power is demonstrated by the consultant through not acknowledging the situation as presented by the nurse; this led to a situation of inter-professional conflict. The doctor ignored the nurse's knowledge of the patient in his coming to a decision. When ordering the sedation to be withheld, he was also failing to acknowledge the nurse's professional and moral obligation to provide patient comfort. In disregarding these fundamental principles in the nursing philosophy and knowledge base, the dominance of medicine's knowledge over nursing was displayed. The power relationship between medicine and nursing was also demonstrated through nursing staff neither questioning nor challenging the medical management plan.

Nurses interpreted the lack of medical consideration for nursing knowledge as an insult to their clinical skills and professional experiences in intensive care. This incident occurred during presentation of a patient on a ward round. The doctor stated:

> 'The patient then had a query arrest [an unconfirmed arrest].' The nurse who had been looking after the patient becomes very defensive and says: 'She had an asystolic arrest and had no output for 2 minutes. We couldn't feel a femoral pulse and she was apnoeic – we rescussed her. By the time the team reached us, she was coming back.' The Consultant says: 'OK' and the round continues. The nurse is still annoyed afterwards – she comes to talk to me. *'I know she had an arrest. There were four nurses there for God's sake. She had no output, she wasn't breathing. We started CPR and put out a call. There was one nurse doing CPR. One maintaining the airway, one feeling for a pulse – and I have to justify to a doctor that she was asystolic. I just feel like saying, look why am I having to go through this with you – she had an asystolic arrest that responded to adrenaline. Really, after all my years of training and experience.'*

Nurses were educated and trained to manage such clinical situations. The nursing distress demonstrated here was not from dealing with the medical emergency, but as result of the nurse having to justify her statement. Such incidents not only served to re-enforce nursing beliefs about the power of medical knowledge, but highlight further potential for conflict within the team.

Power and roles: nursing on the peripheries

As previously noted, the roles adopted by medicine and nursing in the decision-making process could have worked synchronously through nurses presenting information, medicine making decisions and then nursing implementing the decisions made. As previously highlighted, while there were examples of effective communications, these harmonious relationships did not always occur. As reflected in the example I called 'the Swan saga' at the beginning of this chapter, the main power issues arose from how medicine used its authority to make clinical decisions and how nursing informed decision making in intensive care. Medicine ascribed conflict as arising from nursing questioning medical authority in its role as decision maker. Nursing identified the cause of conflict as arising from lack of medical consideration towards the nursing involvement in informing the decision-making process. The focus on these areas not only provoked strong comment and emotion across all sites, it also diverted attention away from other roles in decision making, and the contribution that these areas made to the total decision-making process.

Despite the importance placed by medicine on team working, this was not demonstrated in an explicitly inclusive interdisciplinary mindset during decision making. Even physical and verbal access into decision-making forums was problematic for nursing:

> The nurse's position during the ward round was more varied. The more vocal nurses made an effort to join the circle that inevitably formed at the end of the bed. One actually said to me as the team was lining up 'See how they all gather round now, it's as if they are sharing a secret.' At times the joining of this circle actually necessitated a prod from the nurses to open up the circle. Another leaned right over a bedside table at an awkward angle to join the circle. Some said 'excuse me' and moved in.

Nursing was therefore physically and politically located on the peripheries of the decision-making forums and gave rise to a common nursing perception that: 'nurses are completely ignored on the round by the doctors – the nurse at the bedside and the nurse in charge *are just not valued.*' The concern and feelings of conflict expressed by many nurses was not about medical authority *per se.* The issue was how medical authority was used, and the effect that this had on the contribution of others. Nurses recognised that functionally there had to be one person to make a decision. The issue for nurses was the ability to contribute to, be respected for, and genuine acknowledgement of the unique perspectives that nurses could bring to decision making. This senior nurse is talking about the effect of this on the nursing team:

> The ward round has strong medical authority. This gets stronger the more junior the nurse. G grades are used to challenging and being more assertive. But the vast majority in this unit are junior. Medical staff will cheerfully override their concerns – and this is a source of friction.

Medicine controlled the decision-making forums and those with other agendas were not always recognised. A discussion between a very assertive and credible nurse and a consultant regarding the management of a particularly sick young girl illustrates this:

> Suddenly at the end of the discussion he [the nurse] found the medical staff walking away with no discussion or any answering of his questions. He said: 'Excuse me, but what about my queries?' The consultant said: 'We'll be back later to bronch. her.' The nurse turned to me, held up his hands and said: '*And that's how it goes here, particularly between nurses and doctors*'.

The nurse had concerns he wanted to raise there and then, not wait until after the round. This situation did not appear to be recognised by doctors, who left the bedside without further discussion. This left the nurse feeling frustrated that nursing issues could only be raised at a time acceptable to medical staff.

The power of medicine in decision making was evident. As one consultant informed me: 'They [managers] can't control intensive care. My clinical colleagues need to express their clinical freedom.' This widely accepted view enabled the agenda of medicine to be paramount. One senior nurse revealed problems encountered within the planning of a new unit:

> Take for example, the planning of the new unit which I think demonstrates it quite well. When we talk about the facilities on the unit, the SHO's on-call room has to have a desk, a separate toilet . . . Then you look at the staff areas and you're fighting for an area, for your nursing staff to have a coffee room. We seem to be fighting every inch of the way to get simple things like lockers for every member of staff.

Medical power and the conflict resulting from its use was not just evident in the relationship between medicine and nursing. Conflict was also in evidence between medicine and health care management. One manager extensively discussed their recent experience in attempting to manage a disciplinary procedure against a doctor. As a result of action taken, the manager had been severely reprimanded by the medical director for becoming involved. In all of the sites, the managers had been involved in disciplinary procedures against nurses, but only this manager had any involvement with disciplinary action against a doctor. In all sites, managers were involved with the nursing appraisal and reviews to some extent, but there was no involvement with medical staff reviews. The managers did not have information about, or access, to medical performance reviews or even medical job descriptions.

Nursing was firmly located within the organisational structure, and subject to rules and regulations associated with this. Medicine did not perceive themselves as a collective group located within the trust structure. Doctors continued to operate and function as autonomous individual practitioners with only professional responsibilities and not constrained by organisational conventions. In this way, the medical power base was absolute over both nursing and general management in the organisation.

The decision-making stage in intensive care

As the fieldwork progressed I became aware of specific events that, by their very nature, held dramatic licence. The formal decision-making forums (ward round, service meetings) occurred within a public and formalised environment where roles were well scripted and rehearsed. This contrasted with the private, informal decision-making forums (corridor and bedside meetings) where 'banter and chat and jokes' were the norm. There were also specific observed situations that had a fundamental theatrical component, as illustrated by the following ward round event:

> The nurse said: 'You said yesterday when we raised it [the possibility of the patient having a tracheostomy] that we would discuss it today, so I'm raising it again.' The consultant replied 'Yes I said we would raise it daily for discussion – consider it discussed.' Consultant laughs and turns away, the nurse looks away.

In the study, specific items of equipment were used almost as props. In this way stethoscopes, bedside curtains, and finance sheets became tools used as part of the decision-making process. This is again most powerfully demonstrated in the following excerpt from observation of a ward round. The junior anaesthetist had been holding the results book and had been standing at the back of the large group of people on the ward round:

> When the [laboratory] results are asked for, the circle moves out to include him in the discussion – this is a very powerful repeated action. Sometimes appears as if there is a tussle as to who is going to hold it [the results book].

I therefore began to explore the possibility of re-framing decision making as located on a stage where key players and events were located. The extended theatrical metaphor of drama, ritual and game has been previously used to understand social life (Goffman 1959; Burns 1972). Goffman's theatrical metaphor was therefore examined as a suitable analytical framework through which to gain a different sociological understanding of decision making in intensive care. This section examines how re-reading the field notes in the context of the sociological literature provided an alternative lens with which to view the data. The concept of 'the stage' was therefore used to provide a theoretical and analytical understanding for this work.

Re-reading Goffman's original work together with other sociological accounts that have used this approach (Atkinson 1981; Sinclair 1997) enabled the key regions of the stage: the official front stage, the official back stage, the unofficial front stage, and the unofficial back stage to be described. Despite the fact that there is not a wealth of work that has applied this approach, there are commonalities in the approach taken and the descriptions used; consensus definitions have been used in its application here. The field notes were then re-read and each decision-making forum then located onto one of the four stage regions.

The ward round and the formal operational and business service planning meetings occurred on the front stage. The official front stage area was identified as the region where different social roles were played out through real performances in front of an audience of peers, other team members and the patient/family. This was the high profile setting for decision making where the major players were visible, the scripts most carefully crafted and the roles most clearly defined. In this study, this region was the location of decision-making forums where matters of great drama (life and death of the patient, and of the service) were centre stage, and 'in public'. The unit and trust business meetings were also located on the official front stage, due to the nature of the decision-making issues discussed and the clarity of roles and scripts used.

On the official back stage area of decision making, the meetings between doctors and nurses, without an audience were located. The informal one-to-one discussions regarding patient management on the unit occurred within this region. The official backstage area was defined as the area where impressions meant for the front stage were constructed. The 'hidden' back stage work was undertaken away from the audience, in preparation to meet the front stage requirements. The official back stage was where the rehearsal for decision making occurred. This included getting to know the script through the medical and nursing handovers used to identify the patient management decision-making problems. Back stage work was the area where work was undertaken to ensure that the front stage ran smoothly. This therefore included any type of support work carried out by nursing and medicine to enable front stage decision making to occur. Back stage work also included team and staff meetings that occurred informally, but which were essential to develop and disseminate clinical service decision making. The informal, spontaneous business meetings between nurses, managers and doctors to discuss local service provision (which in turn fed into the front stage management meetings) were also located on this region of the decision-making stage.

Unofficial decision-making strategies, used to direct the decision-making agenda whilst on the front stage, were located on the unofficial front stage. This included the unrecognised decision-making activities undertaken by both nursing and medicine that occurred in the public view. It was the area where decision making occurred on the front stage, but by players not normally considered to have this particular script or role. Without the acclaimed role or script, the decisions made had no recognised authority and were therefore not acknowledged. This included, for example, nursing decisions on administering fluids. Although there were no particular decision-making forums within which this unrecognised decision-making activity occurred, it was more evident through specific behaviours and roles, as will be explored.

The unofficial back stage and lay world areas were not mapped in this study. The unofficial back stage would have included private coffee room discussions and, as previously outlined, I chose not to use that particular data source in this study. In addition, the lay world, including non-health professionals outside of intensive care, was not directly explored in this study on decision making between medicine and nursing. Once the key decision-making forums identified in the study had been located on the decision-making stage, this was represented diagrammatically (Figure 8.1). The decision-making stage, as presented here, provides the basic framework used to develop an alternative analytical perspective on decision making. The metaphorical framework provided a sound setting for the findings of this research, with the regions of the stage providing a comfortable fit with all of the decision-making forums apparent from the data. Application of the dramaturgical perspective highlighted the presumption that the key decision-making forums are located on the front stage region, but that decision-making activity involving doctors and nurses also occurs within other less public, less formal and less officially recognised areas of the decision-making stage.

This book so far has demonstrated that specific areas of knowledge and roles were used in clinical decision making. The field notes were therefore re-read to see if the areas of knowledge and roles could also be located onto the decision-making stage. To validate this process, the data relating to specific decision-making forums, and associated knowledge and roles utilised were re-visited. This allowed the decision-making stage to be redrawn. Figure 8.1 represents knowledge for, and roles in clinical decision making as mapped onto the official front stage, the official back stage, and the unofficial front stage

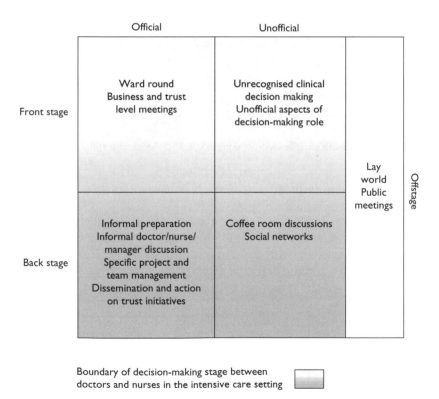

Figure 8.1 The clinical decision-making stage

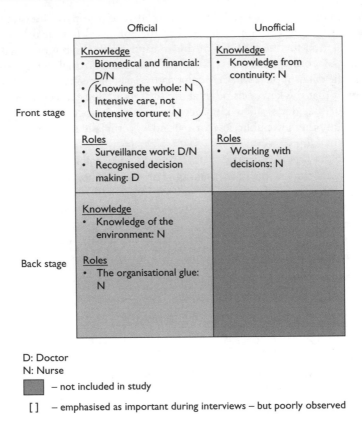

D: Doctor
N: Nurse

▮ – not included in study

[ ] – emphasised as important during interviews – but poorly observed

Figure 8.2 The intensive care decision-making stage: knowledge and roles

regions. The predominant group(s) using, or demonstrating the knowledge and roles are indicated on the diagram.

Through undertaking this procedure, it was clearly demonstrated that on the official front stage, scientific and objective knowledge was key in the biomedical and financial frameworks for decision making. Knowledge resulting from knowing the family and the person in intensive care and from the ethical perspective of intensive care treatment ('Intensive care not intensive torture') was also acknowledged although not as explicitly used. In Figure 8.2 these are therefore placed in brackets. The predominant roles in the decision-making forums on this part of the stage were evident through the recognised authority of medicine to make decisions and the surveillance work undertaken by both nursing and medicine.

The official back stage of decision making was the location for the informal preparation, and later for and the implementation of decision making: in this way, the official front stage objectives could be met and the intensive care milieu could operate smoothly. The key decision-making knowledge used on this area of the stage was knowledge of the environment. This was utilised by both medicine and nursing, but mainly by nursing. The role adopted on this area of the stage was that of acting as the organisational glue for the system. This required knowledge and management of the resources (technological and environmental) in intensive care. It was accepted that these resources were available and needed co-ordinating in order to provide patient care and a clinical service, but the knowledge and skills of how to do this were not fully recognised. This was the back stage and often hidden work that occurred on the decision-making stage, and it was usually nurses that undertook this function.

The unofficial front stage region represented the area where those with no recognised authority made decisions in the 'public arena'. In this work, it was the area where unofficial patient and service management decisions were made. It mainly included the unrecognised decisions made by nurses, who were making the decisions without the formal authority to do so. These were not widely recognised by medicine or, to some extent, by nurses. The knowledge informing these actions was drawn from experience of the environment. Through this, awareness of patient and unit history was used to direct, and influence decision making. Through working with the decisions in this region, the nurse was able to identify and work flexibly with the limitations placed by the decision making. This role enabled the whole system to function more effectively and not become overloaded with demands for decision and action. As indicated in Chapter 7, it was the area where nursing resourcefulness could have the greatest impact on the patient, and nursing inflexibility could be most detrimental to the organisation of clinical and service work.

From this analysis, the dominant knowledge and roles used for front stage decision making are made clear. It is significant that both nursing and medicine have a part to play in this area, but the official front stage remains dominated by medicine. Nurses operate predominantly on other areas of the stage. In this, the official back stage and unofficial front stage activities undertaken by nurses in intensive care fail to be acknowledged or are poorly utilised, and therefore remain invisible in the decision-making process.

Power and conflict on the decision-making stage

The core story of power and conflict has been woven throughout the previous chapters concerning knowledge for, and roles in decision making. As indicated through previous discussion, the nature of this inter-linking is complex and intricate. This section explores the key findings related to power and conflict in interdependent decision making in the context of the data and the literature.

This work has demonstrated that the power held by medicine is instrumental in affecting the nursing decision-making role in intensive care. As a result of the dominant medical knowledge base and role used in decision making, the main nursing contribution for both clinical and service provision was not located in the powerful, public front stage. Nursing work, as summarised in Figure 8.3, predominantly occurred in the unofficial and back stage areas required to enable the decision-making process to operate smoothly. In Figure 8.3, the boundaries of the stage regions have been re-drawn to illustrate the main areas of the stage on which nurses were active in the decision-making process. Nurses did not have a high front stage profile and their total contribution was not recognised by medicine or managers – nor by nursing.

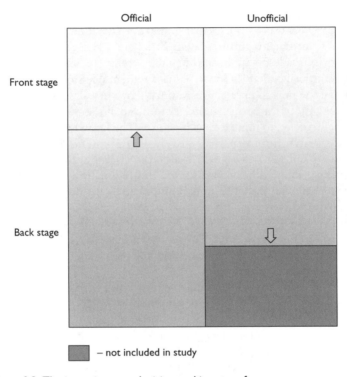

Figure 8.3 The intensive care decision-making stage for nurses

Nurses were therefore a marginalised group in decision making. In order for nurses to input into either clinical management or service management, nurses in the study spoke of the need to understand and 'play the game' of that forum. Through this, nurses had to conform to the norms and values of medicine and of managers, the dominant cultures in decision making. Nursing could then find a place as an agenda item. Whilst this procedure obscured the identity and culture of nursing, without such a manoeuvre there was minimal opportunity for nurses to contribute to decision making.

Nurses were therefore socialised to appreciate more than their worldview (Minh-Ha 1991). This was not so of medicine. Throughout the field data, there were few tangible examples of medical staff truly understanding a nurse's worldview. Street (1992) challenges this imitation of medicine by nurses. She calls for nurses to move beyond the duplication of medicine and to resist medical hegemony. This opposition could be achieved through challenging the process of decision making, rather than challenging the basis on which decisions are made. As Freidson (1970, p. 336) highlighted, there can be agreement that a road is best built by an engineer, 'but whether it should be built at all, and where it should be located are not wholly esoteric questions'.

Nurses were not obviously present, or did not have clear access to the official front decision-making stage; nurses did not contribute to decision-making agendas on their own terms. As has been detailed, nursing issues only gained access to the front stage when synchronised with wider organisational or government concerns (Rafferty 1992). The success of any challenge by nurses to organisational or medical hegemony rested on the ability of nurses to adapt or assimilate their view of nursing to that of the decision-maker's vision of the health service. Nursing therefore remains in a similar position as described by Robinson and Strong (1987) some time ago.

Nurses spoke of conflicts with medicine at the bedside with nursing colleagues or in the coffee room: in areas that nurses considered private spaces (Liaschenko 1998), areas of their own. These conversations often made use of the vocabulary of complaint (Turner 1986), revealing the frustrations of nurses whose professional voice was being restricted by medical and bureaucratic structures. Although the results of this study are similar to Porter's work (1991, 1995), they contrast with Hughes's work (1988) where there was open dissent from nursing staff about medical staff. Alternative readings of Hughes's work (Porter 1998) may illuminate grounds for this difference.

A key rationale directing the initial sample sites was to ascertain what impact specific nursing developments, for example nursing diagnosis and nursing development units, had on how medicine and nursing work together. This study has demonstrated that in the context of intensive care, such nursing initiatives do not appear to expand the contribution of nursing to decision making with doctors. There was evidence of increased nursing knowledge of the patient and commitment to team working issues, but if such sources of knowledge were not used within team working or if interdisciplinary meetings were not supported by medicine, then such efforts did not influence patient or unit outcome. Such patient-focused approaches may enhance the nursing role in independent nursing activities, but do not necessarily improve the ways in which medicine and nursing work together.

Nurses in the field were unable to articulate the total contribution made by nurses across all regions of the decision-making stage. It continued to be the front stage activities that were the most recognised and afforded the highest status. However, nursing dissatisfaction was not driven by a need to become more centre stage, but to have acknowledgement and recognition of the unofficial and back stage work undertaken. In analysing the challenge made by nursing on medical autonomy, nursing's motives were not to overthrow medicine, but to re-negotiate and reform traditional patterns of subordination (Light 1993). This is an important issue as, unless the total nursing contribution is recognised by all, nursing will remain invisible in the health care arena and nursing's value will go unrecognised.

The visibility of such alternative and complementary areas of nursing knowledge and roles within the health care team was a key issue raised within this study. Recognition of these non-medical areas have been seen as pivotal to claiming legitimate independence from medicine (Walby and Greenwall 1994), but in this study its importance was to claim effective interdependence between nursing and medicine.

Strategies to make the invisible, visible

Despite the focus of this chapter on power and conflict in intensive care, there was evidence that medicine and nursing recognised the need to work together. Medical and nursing staff interviewed had an awareness of the conflict and frustrations experienced in the decision-making process. From this, both medicine and nursing were able to highlight practice changes to enable a more collaborative approach. It was clear that medicine and nursing saw a shared responsibility for this.

Nurses were cognisant of that fact that whilst there were traditional power issues to be addressed, nurses could be active partners in working towards resolution of this situation. It was well accepted by the senior nursing staff that: nurses don't always make the best of the opportunities to present themselves. All study sites encouraged and supported deliberative behaviour changes in nursing staff to enable a greater nursing contribution to be made in this area. One senior nurse discusses this:

> The challenge is how we are all going to agree. How we are going to work together when we have different agendas . . . It is just accepted that we work by different rules . . . We work with a different set of values and agendas. Different mechanisms of how to deal with it – of negotiation, of getting what we say as valued . . . I think it's important to look at how we develop our staff.

Such developing strategies were primarily concerned with the personal and interpersonal development. Through such development, it was anticipated that nursing staff could be more active in the decision-making process and work more effectively with medicine.

It was acknowledged by all that credible clinical experience was vital to achieve input into decision making. This was used as a source of knowledge and experience to validate what the issues were, and when to raise them. As highlighted by one nurse:

But you need to build yourself up, for example if you want your input into the ward round – you need to time your input, not just necessarily wait for the end – to choose the most appropriate time. And to do this, you use your knowledge, what has worked in the past, what other patients have you cared for and how can you use that knowledge to get your concerns noted. To break through that inner circle at the end of the bed. You know, doctors huddle together in their little circle and it's like you cannot break into that, but you have to, you have to be able to raise your issues and to have input into the ward round.

The issue of confidence was clearly and repeatedly articulated as an attribute enabling contribution to decision making. As raised by this nurse:

The role of the nurse at the bedside tends to be very much part of the ward round when looking after their patient – but unless they are confident and senior enough to speak up they may not always represent their patient . . . There are some nurses where if they have an issue to raise, they will not let the ward round move on until they have raised that issue.

Nurses therefore responded in diverse ways to this challenge. Under-confident nurses were generally more passive, whereas more confident and experienced staff adopted a more proactive role in decision making. The following excerpt demonstrates one such passive approach:

The consultant asks if the patient has had an ECG. Everyone looks blank and no reply is elicited. The consultant then turns to the nurse 'Has he had an ECG? The nurse replies: 'No not yet.' The consultant asks: 'Right then, can we do one?' They then turn their backs to the nurse and consultant says: 'We'll be back later.' There was no opportunity, nor did the nurse make it, for any further discussion. After the ward round left, the nurse made the comment: 'Why should I bother doing this if they're not going to look at it.'

The medical request for information is made, and a passive nursing response given. The nurse does not agree that the information is going to be used in patient management and yet does not challenge this medical decision.

At other times, not only did the nurse identify the problem through information giving, but also gave a possible solution together with a rationale. This was then presented for discussion and decision making. The following is typical of this situation, where a doctor and nurse are discussing a patient with continuing low blood pressure. The nurse begins:

Well I wonder if floating a Swan would help? At least we'd know what the optimal pressures were and if we needed to manipulate her afterload.

Perhaps she needs volume because she's going septic. I mean, we are kinda expecting it aren't we? Doctor:Yes, I see what you mean . . . I'm starting to agree with your suggestion now.

In this field example, the role of the person raising and clarifying the decision-making issue also had the potential effect of influencing the decision made. This was an approach noted in the more experienced staff. It was more likely to occur on a one-to-one basis, than in a large formal decision-making forum. Confidence was associated with being able to speak up within large inter-disciplinary forums, one within which nurses did not anticipate others would necessarily support their suggestions.

A further key strategy supported by all experienced nurses concerned the nurse's behaviour during the ward round. The complex milieu of intensive care made many demands on the bedside nurse. Less experienced nursing staff used the routinisation of work to ensure that all facets of care were attended to. Junior nurses in intensive care worked in a very controlled way. Although the carrying out of hourly patient observations gave important structure to their work, it could detract from input into decision making. This senior nurse noted:

> The nurses are always doing distracting things, like emptying urine bags, ferreting under the bed, fiddling with the bed pedals. The novice works in a more structured way – oh the 08.00 obs are due – I must do those. We should work in a more loose way, oh the ward round is here, and I'll do the obs later. Sometimes everyone's there and standing with their back to you – I'll just put my elbows out and say 'excuse me' to sometimes, just out of devilry, I'll stand in the middle of the circle, in front of everyone! The nurse needs to be clear of the plan for the day, cos you know that you're not going to find a doctor for hours.

The need for nurses to present themselves to the ward round, to make and take opportunities to become involved in decision making, was strongly asserted. The aim of developing nursing staff was to enable them to prioritise care so that attendance at the decision-making forums became a priority. While there were no direct references to similar strategies being adopted during service decision making, a more proactive and assertive stance was used by all the experienced nurses involved at this level of service management. The following extract from a senior nurse demonstrates this most strongly:

> You need to be assertive, sometimes you can see they [doctors and managers] are being condescending – yes, yes, because she functions well in other ways we'll let her have her foibles. Doctors have no understanding where nurses are coming from. They are crisp, white and clean, the new types do talk about emotions, but basically they expect to be listened to.

When they talk – you have to play their game. Consultants have a big ego. If you look at the advanced practice role – that's what its all about – power and role. As a senior nurse, I also have an ego. I have worked very hard to get where I am, I therefore expect to be consulted.

In recognising the importance of being present for decision-making discussions, senior nurses recognised the value they could have acting as role models. The role of the nurse in charge could assist the bedside nurse by undertaking essential care, and therefore allowing the bedside nurse to attend decision-making forums. As highlighted by one senior nurse:

They [nurses] don't help themselves, they are very often doing the obs. And have their back to the ward round. I see it as the role of the [nurse] co-ordinator to push the nurse forward. For example if the nurse is doing something, I will go over and take over so that she will get to the round.

In all the units, there was an established practice that involved the nurse in charge speaking with each bedside nurse before the ward round to identify and rehearse issues to be raised on the ward round. This also enabled the nurse in charge to actively support the bedside nurse, if required.

The more experienced nurses consciously developed an awareness of the competing agendas, either in the clinical or service arena. This was then used by nurses to guide how decision-making issues were broached: 'You need to play games with the managers and the doctors – to know what each of them wants. You don't do anything different, just differently. You need to be more pro-active and think how to respond to the different personalities and the different agendas.' Through this, subtle covert measures were taken by nurses to influence decision making.

Medicine espoused the rhetoric of team work and the importance of the contribution of nursing. Doctors were aware of the frustrations arising from team working, but took little responsibility for this situation. The following excerpt from a consultant interview highlights this issue:

I think that our working relationships are very forward – we are all part of the team – if the doctor isn't there it fails, and if the nurse isn't there, it fails . . . I think we [doctors] lead the team by involvement and motivation. We promote, motivate, demonstrate respect, and call each other by first names. I think that some of the nurses may feel that there is a hierarchy, but I think that it's their problem. *They're shit scared of medicine, but that's their problem.* The junior staff [junior doctors] have a rough ride if they don't know the patient. They are trained by embarrassment. Nursing is different, it's high on *mollycoddling*. Nurses appreciate hand holding.

Medicine made it clear that resolution of any teamwork problems lay within the domain of nursing. This supports previous empirical work (Prescott and

Bowen 1985; Baggs *et al.* 1992) and gives further evidence that medical and nursing staff hold different beliefs about the nature of collaborative working.

In the field, medical staff pointed to the fact that nurses were present at decision-making forums (clinical or service) and assumed that this fact alone attested to medicine's valuing nursing. The only concrete strategy highlighted by medicine that enabled nursing to contribute to decision-making forums was through medical staff giving nurses the opportunity to raise their concerns at the end of the discussion. There was no attempt at identification of ways to better utilise other areas of nursing knowledge or nursing role within intensive care.

It was within nursing that strategies had been developed to address the conflict arising in decision making in intensive care. These approaches were fundamentally behavioural, concerning the nature of interaction with medicine. The strategies were focused on developing the developmental and assertiveness skills of the nurse, and not on challenging the very basis of the decision-making itself. This is entirely consistent with the solutions offered by Stein (1967; Stein *et al.* 1990) that have been previously highlighted.

Despite the vociferous statements made by medical and nursing in private spaces, there were few examples of open conflict in the field. As demonstrated in previous chapters, potential areas of conflict were managed or negotiated, predominantly by the nursing staff. This is an example of negotiated order that has already been explored through Svensson (1996) and Allen's (1997) work. Through such actions, nursing acquiesced with the medical agenda, and did not directly challenge the position of the nursing knowledge base or role. Nursing's power was used to manage the division of labour and reduce conflict between medicine and nursing. This did not directly address the key structural issues at the root cause of the conflict and acted to endorse rather than contest the dominance of the existing power base.

Nursing and medicine often presented two extreme and contrasting positions in this study. However, the importance of understanding each other's point of view was one that was frequently raised and spoken of as 'a two-way thing'. This was seen as important so that mutual goals and agendas could be set and worked to, otherwise as one nurse commented: 'What's the point? If medicine is running one race, and nursing another – they may as well shut the unit.' Nonetheless, there was little shared understanding of some of the most basic issues. Even the organisation of the medical and nursing day, and the timing of the rounds were sources of frustration: 'At the end of the ward round, all the doctors went for coffee. There appeared to be no allocation or organisation, which required nurses hunting for the doctors who were looking after their patient if there was a problem. One nurse commented: "They just can't get themselves organised, there is no patient allocation and no time management."' This was contrasted in an interview with a consultant: 'I'm ready for the ward round, and what happens, at 09.15 all the nurses go on their break. There is absolutely no concept to be at the beds for the ward round. I'm not saying it's their faults. It's all our faults.' In reality, the vision of one race being run had not been realised.

Concluding thoughts

This study has demonstrated that medical knowledge and roles remain the most discernible aspects of the decision-making process. The visibility of alternative and complementary areas of nursing knowledge and roles within the health care team is less evident. As previously stated, the recognition of these non-medical areas has been used to claim legitimate independence from medicine. Here these areas have been used to claim effective interdependence between nursing and medicine.

Both medicine and nursing were aware of the power and conflict within decision making. Medicine has ultimate authority and accountability in the decision-making process. Nursing perceives itself to have reduced power with which to influence and inform decision making. Medicine ascribes this to the subordinate position that nursing perceives themselves in; nursing believes that this subordination is continually re-enforced by medicine.

The historical drive for nursing to achieve professional status has not been instrumental in achieving nursing visibility within health care decision making. The literature does reveal some alternative options through which nursing can make its expertise visible, and directly challenge the structural restraints imposed by medicine and the organisation. The mobilisation of nursing's collective power and the use of occupational strategies (Salvage 1988) together with the endorsement of a patient-centred, holistic model of health may enable greater occupational control and practitioner autonomy. It may more directly challenge traditional doctor–nurse relationships (Witz 1992).

Davies (1996, pp. 149–150) calls for a dislodging of the gendered model of professionalism and the establishment of a new practitioner in health care who is 'neither autonomous nor passive, but interdependent'. Although current government policy indicates a move towards this vision, successful implementation of such a patient-focused model to date seems to result from individual and local encouragement rather than cultural and whole-system support.

Chapter 9

Breaking through the inner circle

Rhetoric or reality?

An important moment for me during the study fieldwork came when nursing staff were describing one of their perceptions about the ward round. This was encapsulated in the phrase 'Breaking through the inner circle'. The words aptly described the spatial tensions occurring in the ward round, and summarised the experiences of nursing staff in their aim to contribute to clinical decision making. It represented the situation where medicine and nursing operated within their own domains, and how it was principally nurses who sought to influence medicine in order to re-define care delivery. This phrase became symbolic and, therefore, is used in the title of this book, and as the heading for this last chapter. In the chapter, I summarise the key themes to emerge from the book, and explore the implications of this work. Present and future opportunities will be considered that may enable a working environment for collaborative practice to be attained. However, this can only be achieved if the inner circles are breached and the territorial boundaries across the health care teams are broken down.

I will first present some limitations of this book. In contributing to the sociological literature, this book indirectly explores both structure and agency. I have not explored the precise nature of the inter-relationship between the macro and micro sociological level of analysis. Whilst structural components of interdependent decision making, with the influence of social structure theories, and agency issues with use of social action theories, have been described, the mechanism of the interaction between the two was not examined in detail. Layder (1998, p. 99) asserts that a multidimensional approach, acknowledging the diversity of social reality, is required: 'Methodologically, therefore, it is necessary to find ways of weaving them [structure and agency] together while preserving their integrity as distinct, but relatively autonomous, from each other.' In future work, this particular aspect will need greater consideration and more explicit consideration within both methodological debate and empirical work.

Throughout the fieldwork, I was profoundly surprised by the frankness of expression, especially from the medical staff. This led to concerns regarding the validity of data from this source. My concerns were that they were either delivering a 'cultural script' (Silverman 1993, p. 96), or managing self-presentation in the interview, or fabricating tales so that the facts remained concealed (Denzin 1970). I had to view the interviews as either 'true' reports or as situated narratives. Medical staff interviews had a recurring pattern concerning attitudes towards nursing with strongly opinionated standpoints. In contrast, nursing staff interviews demonstrated an alternative, but also repetitive, pattern representing the nursing response towards medicine (the atrocity tales). The approach adopted during the analysis of these accounts was consistent with Baruch's moral tales (1982). The findings from the interviews were therefore not treated as either right or wrong, but used as accounts to evidence the underlying issues.

Critics of this work may believe that my findings appear to build on recognised stereotypical patterns of behaviour between doctors and nurses, and that this book presents the antitheses of harmonious working relationships. Indeed, this work may be read in a way as to reinforce the status quo, rather than seeking to promote new ways of working. I would like to make several points here. First, the focus in this book was on one area only, that of clinical decision making: other domains of interdependent working were not explored and might have yielded very different data. Second, the data excerpts used in this book were representative of the field evidence. The excerpts represent the reality in those units for doctors and nurses at that time. Finally, it is important to note that neither medicine nor nursing is a homogeneous group, but comprises a diverse range of individuals, with a range of personal and professional characteristics. In the field there were examples of strongly collaborative medical and nursing staff, and also of those who were obstructive and defensive in interactions with their colleagues. The discussion issues raised in this book were based on the analysis of collective – rather than individual – positions. The attempt is to represent the reality of the clinical practice coalface. I believe it is from this point that realistic goal setting and planning can be undertaken in order to strive towards more effective team working.

Breaking through the inner circle: the core story

Intensive care decision making continues to be strongly driven by the knowledge and roles held by medicine. Clinical decision making involving doctors and nurses is controlled by medical power as nursing does not, in the main, hold a recognised authority in decision making. This results in medicine (and management) setting the agenda for clinical decision making, and directing the specific areas of decisions to be made.

Different sources of knowledge are used in the decision-making process. There are areas of knowledge which are used by both medicine and nursing, for example patient response to drug therapy. There are other areas of knowledge, which are acknowledged by medicine, but held and used predominantly by nursing. These include the areas of knowledge consistent with nursing's holistic, person-centred philosophy of care with interpersonal and ethical issues in care.

Nursing holds specific knowledge for decision making that results from being at the bedside and having a presence on the unit on a continuous basis. Yet, this knowledge is not fully used by medicine in the decision-making process. Nurses also hold extensive reserves of knowledge resulting from their experience of the intensive care environment, and of the specific organisation within which the unit is located. This source of knowledge, intrinsic to the functioning of the unit and the implementation of both patient and service policy, appears to be unacknowledged by medicine, managers and nurses themselves.

The role perceived by both medicine and nursing to hold most power within decision making is that associated with having authority to make clinical decisions: this dominant role is held by medical staff. In contrast, the nurses' role in decision making is primarily concerned with informing the decision-making process, working with the decisions made, and managing the decision-making environment. The nursing role is therefore fundamental to the implementation of the decisions made by doctors. Nurses do make decisions within their role of working with the clinical decisions that are made, but these are largely unrecognised by medical and managerial staff. Neither medical, managerial, nor, at times, nursing staff, value the contribution made by nursing to the decision-making process. Partly because of this, nurses remain unable to identify or unsuccessful in articulating their specific decision-making knowledge and roles.

In undertaking a dramaturgical analysis of decision making in intensive care, the official front stage medical knowledge and roles continue to have the greatest influence. Medicine thus retains its powerful decision-making position. Doctors and managers define the nursing role in decision making by association with medical and managerial aims. Nursing does not therefore exist independently of, or complementary to, medicine. Nursing is defined by medicine, in a way that reinforces the dominant worldview.

In decision-making practice, sources of knowledge and roles that are alternative and complementary to those of medicine, such as those held by nursing, are recognised but not valued. Both the back stage decision-making implementation work and unofficial front stage decision-making activities, undertaken by nursing, fail to be recognised in the decision-making process. Demands for greater input by nurses into the decision making are read by medical staff as nurses wanting greater authority over the process. This is incongruous to nurses, who are essentially seeking recognition of the complementary roles and knowledge they hold and attempting to work towards a more democratic partnership in the decision-making process. Conflict between nursing and medicine subsequently develops due to the frustration of nurses unable to influence and inform decision making, and concern from medical staff about nursing intentions.

Both doctors and nurses espouse the principle of a team approach to intensive care and endorse working towards effective team working in decision making. However, medicine and nursing have different expectations of team working. Specific strategies to achieve collaborative working are mainly undertaken by nurses. These are not meant as a direct challenge to the medical hierarchy of knowledge and roles in decision making, but are intended to focus on the interpersonal development of the nurse to enable greater impact and contribution during decision-making forums.

This work has drawn attention to the nursing knowledge available for decision making, and the nursing role in the total decision-making process. Nurses integrate patient and family points of view into their knowledge base. This is surely consonant with the current concern for a patient-focused health care service (DoH 2000b). This perspective is particularly important in the critical environment of intensive care, where both patient and relatives are vulnerable. Nursing's ability and skill in translating decision making into action through the decision implementation process has also been highlighted. Close observation of patients and of unit activity requires skilful implementation of the decisions made, and constant refinement and evaluation to determine the impact of those decisions. Within this work, nurses at clinical and service levels make unofficial and unrecognised decisions that in turn enable doctors' decisions to be successfully implemented.

It is significant that this work is located within an intensive care environment, an area where nursing roles have now developed to the extent that the boundaries between nursing and medical roles are becoming blurred. Despite the complex skills and knowledge acquired by nurses in this clinical area, nursing's ability to influence and contribute to decision making officially remains restricted and unrecognised. The developed role of the nurse in intensive care has not created a substantial challenge to the traditional medical hierarchy of knowledge or roles. This is an important consideration if the current political agenda of achieving working partnerships is to be addressed in contemporary health care.

Living with uncertainty, not in it

We are living and working in times of great change where there is a balance to be achieved in what is being demanded from health care against the available resources. There has been, and will continue to be, on-going public, political and professional interest in health care workforce issues. The health care labour forces in the various disciplines are, by their very nature, interdependent. Doctors, nurses and other team members do not develop roles in isolation from each other, but as part of a complex and interdependent system. As the core skills and responsibilities of such groups change, the organisation of the health care workforce will become increasingly out of line with the traditional map of health care professions. The changes need careful and sustained whole system planning to be managed effectively. It is anticipated that any resultant change in workforce profiles will not become fully established for at least ten to fifteen years (Parish 2003). This emphasises the complexity of the process of identifying the core of each health care role, redefining what health care work is, and how this could be undertaken. What specific issues can be taken away from this work to help practitioners work with such uncertainty?

Health care has traditionally been defined as medical care (Hancock 1995), and nursing work has gone unrecognised. In this book, I have sought to demonstrate that medical and nursing skills, as perceived by health care practitioners and health care managers, are not commensurable. This book has highlighted the complex and diverse knowledge used and roles adopted by nurses in decision making in intensive care. Through raising awareness of the discrete and interdependent role undertaken by the intensive care nurse, a more expansive framework has been provided to identify the profile and contribution of the intensive care nurse. Unique areas of knowledge and role have been identified that are central to the nurse's contribution to interdependent decision-making development. How these are integrated into the current ethos of evidence-based practice has yet to be fully addressed. This study has contributed to the understanding of the role of the nurse in contemporary health care. Through use of this expanded framework, the increased responsibilities being placed on, and taken up by nurses, can be identified and acknowledged. The framework can then be used so that responsibility can be matched with an appropriate level of authority within a patient-focused culture. It is yet to be demonstrated whether the new pay arrangements (DoH 2002) being introduced will impact on this. However, it is disappointing that the common competency approach that appreciates broader areas of expertise is not being adopted across all health care disciplines.

This book has, importantly, questioned the impact that contemporary nursing role developments (primary nursing, nursing development units) have made on interdependent health care issues. It is clear that settings and specialities within which nurses have historically developed more autonomous and innovative roles are those environments in which medicine had little involvement or had a vested interest in supporting nursing empowerment. The nursing developments encountered in this study, for example primary nursing and nursing development units, were strongly driven by a patient focused philosophy. In this book, the developments were being implemented within an environment where the fundamental nature of relationships within the health care team had not been addressed. The salient issue is that, whilst efforts to improve health care issues remain focused or driven by only one discipline of the team, progress will be limited to within that discipline. Any emerging health and social care systems in the future will depend less on individual practitioners for care and more on the resources offered by the whole health care team; the shift will be from traditional medical-based teams to team-based working (DoH 2003). Therefore if nurses wish to address issues which impact on the interdisciplinary team (nursing contribution to decision making with doctors) then an interdisciplinary approach must be taken.

The different definitions of collaboration used by doctors and nurses have been demonstrated in this text. The conflict arising from such different expectations has also been highlighted through the core story. Until the two worldviews of medicine and nursing are mutually acknowledged and recognised by both doctors and nurses, the resultant conflict will continue. It is unlikely that the vision of the collaborative team presented in current national health policy making (DoH 1999) will be fully realised. The failure to achieve it will reduce the inter-professional effectiveness between nursing and medicine, with the concomitant consequences on the delivery of patient care and on clinical services.

This book has demonstrated that nurses work to achieve an interdependent model of team working through collaboration. To achieve true interdisciplinary, interdependent teams, driven by the local contextual and patient needs, requires the current professional ideology of a unique professional knowledge base to be rescinded, and supportive organisational structures and cultures to be developed. This may require some of the very configurations and processes, for example the ward round, that in their current format militate against teamwork, to be modified to encompass collaborative working practices. It also requires a recognised need for support, development and education of medical staff to work in effective clinical teams.

Nursing aspires to a more equal partnership with medicine in intensive care. Yet it has been demonstrated that medicine does not appear to be active in directly facilitating this. The study demonstrated how a lack of mutual under-standing of collaborative partnerships leads to conflict in interprofessional working. Nursing staff made attempts to influence the structural dominance of medicine's power base through use of strategies directed at improving social interaction. Nurses could, alternatively, consider strategies to make explicit the knowledge and skills contained within the official back stage and unofficial front stage regions. These are potentially powerful, yet unexplored, aspects of the nursing role. For without such role functions, decision implementation and the development of decision making would not exist (Barker 1996). Nursing roles in decision making are not only complementary to medicine, but are also required in order for health care to be delivered. Nursing must realise this, and clearly articulate it, in order to influence the decision-making process.

If the health care power base is to be re-shaped, specific issues will need to be addressed. Doctors (and managers) will need to re-consider nurses' authority to match the increasing nursing responsibility held with the current role developments. Nurses, at an individual and collective level, must consider if this is what they aspire to. Nurses will also need to re-consider issues of account-ability, and be prepared to take on the associated obligations that come with this. If roles are to be redefined, there will need to be clearer exposition of what individual and collective accountability means, and how this is understandable to patients and to health workers alike. This could be through a re-examination of the concept of hierarchical versus multiple accountability: a key concept for flexible working in clinical directorates (Hancock 1995). All parties, including nurses, must be critical of their own practice, and be held accountable for their actions.

This text has not directly addressed nursing's preoccupation with attaining professional status. From this study, it has been intimated that professional status will not immediately affect how medicine responds to nursing. If traditional professional structures are radically reviewed, there may be the development of generic workers within health care. This may, in the current climate, seem inconceivable and requires a dramatic philosophical shift for both doctors and nurses within the health service. The possibility does, though, serve to challenge both nurses and doctors, and to emphasise that nursing and medicine should move away from debates on professional status, and concentrate on becoming a skilled public service serving the patient.

In recognising the need to challenge traditional power bases directly, the current government solution is restricted to the observation that all disciplines have a role in addressing this (DoH 1997, 2000a, 2000b). In the NHS Plan, it is clearly stated that, by 2004, the majority of NHS staff will be working under agreed protocol. However, there is no specific reference made as to how medical work will change and medicine's use of protocol-driven care is not reviewed. Whilst acknowledging the political complexity of the situation, a stronger challenge could be made to medicine. There is a clearly a responsibility at local clinical level to influence traditional working practices and behaviours, but equally the challenge must also come from the government, leading professional bodies, chief executives and trust medical directors. The importance of the regulatory bodies and professional associations in providing national leadership to overcome local barriers to change is important. It remains imperative that all parties take an active role in working towards a team-focused approach.

The culture is changing, as demonstrated through the publication of radical discussion documents (BMA 2002; IPPR 2002), and evidence of interdisciplinary and shared learning (Cray 1989). Learning in groups can be an effective way to effect performance and behavioural change in groups. This study has identified the areas of knowledge held by doctors and nurses as being important for intensive care. Taking a strong interdisciplinary approach, through well facilitated case conferences, seminars and clinical courses, will enable doctors and nurses to understand such different knowledge bases and expertise. This could be achieved through shared and integrated learning (Ross and Mackenzie 1996). Both doctors and nurses need to be educated to listen to, reflect on and value each others' voices. This may include greater use of interdisciplinary meetings to discuss clinical and service issues in order to gradually increase awareness, within the team, of individuals' roles and knowledge.

The recently introduced concept of clinical governance (DoH 1998) with its accountability framework for quality improvements, may provide one strategy for enabling nurses to contribute more effectively to decision-making development, and provide medical staff with a means of comprehending complementary sources of knowledge and expertise. Clinical governance makes explicit an agenda for clinical partnerships with greater importance on interprofessional working (NHSE 1999). Through this approach, nurses and doctors would be seen as partners in decision making, a position that was not revealed in this study. This structure may make more clear the professional and organisational role, responsibilities and expertise encompassed within health care roles.

A further strategy may be to promote an expanded conceptualisation of decision making within health care. Evaluation of health care decision making has traditionally been dominated by outcome evaluation. The debate on health sector reforms has concentrated on the content and outcomes of policy, to the detriment of the actors, processes and decision-making context (Walt and Gilson 1994). There is a need to explore the central issue of power held by all health care actors at national and local levels, together with the resultant implications for the health service. This will require a methodology capable of capturing dynamic organisational aspects. Through this, other issues concerning informing and implementing decision making will be made more transparent. Both nurses and doctors will need to develop and be educated into appreciating the unique, yet complementary, roles and knowledge that each brings to the decision-making process. Nurses will be required to articulate their knowledge and assert their contribution to policy, and medicine will be required to realise this: all must play a part in the process.

Health care decision making can result in reactive or proactive responses (Hennessy and Spurgeon 2000). I suggest that nurses need to develop more proactive responses within decision making. Nurses need to understand fully the nursing consequences of a particular decision-making initiative. Nurses need to be proactive in their response to decision making and to illustrate how, as a collective body, they can influence health care policy. There has been a long-standing socialisation process that has established the traditional working practices between medicine and nursing. If nurses are passive in the decision-making process, and their discontentment with this situation is leading to conflict, then nurses must take some responsibility for addressing the problem. Nurses could usefully contribute to decision making through the challenging of clinical practices and financial constraints, providing of alternative service options, and interpreting user needs (Pursey and Brocklehurst 1996).

Hancock (1995) believes that nurses have more influence in the health care services than they realise. The future of the developing nursing role and of advancing practice in intensive care lies with nurses realising the potential in developing collaborative partnerships and reconsidering interdependency. The future of the nursing role in decision making lies with nurses realising the inherent power through the complementary decision-making role that nurses take relative to medicine. The fundamental use of this power must be to increase influence on the politically determined practices of the day in order to improve patient services: not to increase the professional power of nurses and nursing *per se*.

The epilogue

Collaboration is a testing concept for all health care practitioners. It requires respect and trust for oneself and others, and a sharing of information and power: values that have not traditionally been demonstrated within health care relationships. Adopting a collaborative approach in health care mandates all team members, including medical and nursing staff, to reflect critically on attitudes and behaviours. In any relationship there is always the potential for the abuse of power over others. Nurses must take their share of responsibility in this and the question must be raised whether nurses have taken advantage of their own power base over patients or other health care professionals. Nursing's seeking to explore its own identity must not become a preoccupation with exclusivity and independence, to the extent of failing to acknowledge the contribution of others. Such an omission would not add any value to the development of effective working relationships with others.

In a health care climate that aims to foster a philosophy of clinical governance, all intensive care practitioners must engage in developing not only local clinical policy, but also national service frameworks: becoming partners in health care policy. This will require an essential shift in the organisational culture, a feat only to be achieved through real commitment from all staff to work towards accountability, team work and collaboration. This culture will require that all expertise and roles required in intensive care be acknowledged, in order for the contribution of all team members to be recognised.

Intensive care, by its very nature, mandates a team approach where all disciplines are required to contribute effectively to care. However, the skills and knowledge once owned by medicine are now integrated into the everyday practice of nursing, encompassed within the delivery of holistic and humanistic care. This has led to an increasing emphasis on nursing identity and practitioner autonomy. I believe we now need to move beyond a preoccupation with concepts like 'uniqueness' and 'independence' within intensive care, to address the fundamental interdependent nature of working relationships within the intensive care team.

Mutually respectful working partnerships, based on acknowledgement of the discrete professional knowledge and roles that contribute to the total care, must be cultivated and maintained. It is only when we discard professional tribalisms and behave supportively, not destructively, to others and ourselves that effective working alliances can be engendered. I believe that the future of intensive care will emerge from a consensus of the knowledge and the roles held by all practitioners in this field: the uniqueness of this will lie in that consensus.

References

Abbott, A. (1988) *The Systems of Professions: An Essay on the Division of Expert Labour.* University of Chicago Press, Chicago.

Ackroyd, S. (1996) Traditional and new management in the NHS hospital service and their effects on nursing. In *Themes and Perspectives in Nursing.* 2nd edn. Soothill, K., Henry, C. and Hendrick, K. eds. Chapman and Hall, London.

Adams, A., Lugsden, E., Chase, J., Arber, S. and Bond, S. (2000) Skill-mix changes and work intensification in nursing. *Work, Employment and Society,* 14: 541–555.

Adamson, B. J., Kenny, D. T. and Wilson-Barnett, J. (1995) The impact of perceived medical dominance on the workplace satisfaction of Australian and British nurses. *Journal of Advanced Nursing,* 21: 172–183.

Adler, P. and Adler, P. (1987) *Membership Roles in Field Research.* Sage Publications, Newbury Park, CA.

Agar, M. H. (1980) *The Professional Stranger: An Informal Introduction to Ethnography.* Sage Publications, Newbury Park, CA.

Alaszewski, A. (1995) Restructuring health and welfare professions in the United Kingdom. In *Health Professions and the State in Europe.* Johnson, T., Larkin, G. and Saks, M., eds. Routledge, London.

Alavi, C. and Cattoni, J. (1995) Good nurse, bad nurse. *Journal of Advanced Nursing,* 21: 231–260.

Alder, P. A. and Alder, P. (1987) Observation techniques. In *Handbook of Qualitative Research.* Denzin, N. K. and Lincoln, Y. S., eds. Sage Publications, Thousand Oaks.

Alford, R. R. (1975) *Health Care Politics.* University of Chicago Press, Chicago.

Allen, D. (1997) The nursing medicine boundary: negotiated order. *Sociology of Health and Illness,* 19, 4: 498–520.

Allen, D. (2001) *The Changing Shape of Nursing Practice: The Role of Nurses in the Hospital Division of Labour.* Routledge, London.

Alpert, H. B. (1992) Gryzmish – towards an understanding of collaboration. *Nursing Clinics of North America,* 27: 47–59.

Alt-White, A. C., Charns, M. and Strayer, R. (1983) Personal, organisational and managerial factors related to nurse–physician collaboration. *Nursing Administration Quarterly,* 8: 8–18.

Anderson, J. (1984) *Public Policy Making.* 3rd edn. CNS College Publishing, New York.

Anderson, J. and O'Brien, M. (1995) Challenges for the future: the nurses role in weaning patients from mechanical ventilation. *Intensive and Critical Care Nursing*, 11, 1: 2–5.

Annandale, E. (1996) Working on the front line: risk culture and nursing in the new NHS. *Sociological Review*, 44, 3: 416–451.

Anspach, R. R. (1993) *Deciding who lives: fateful choices in the Intensive Care Nursery.* University of California Press, Berkeley.

Antrobus, S. (1995) Teachers play the triangle. *Nursing Management*, 1, 9: 12–13.

Ashworth, P. (1990) High technology and humanity for intensive care. *Intensive and Critical Care Nursing*, 6: 150–160.

Atkinson, P. (1981, 1997) *The Clinical Experience: The Construction and Reconstruction of Medical Reality.* Gower, Farnborough.

Atkinson, P. (1995) *Medical Talk and Medical Work.* Sage Publications, London.

Atkinson, P. and Hammersley, M. (1994) Ethnography and participant observation. In *Handbook of Qualitative Research.* Denzin, N. K. and Lincoln, Y. S., eds. Sage, Thousand Oaks, C.A.

Audit Commission (1995) *The Doctor's Tale.* Audit Commission, HMSO, London.

Audit Commission (1999) *Critical to Success: The Place of Efficient and Effective Critical Care Services within the Acute Hospital.* Audit Commission, London.

Baggs, J. G. (1994) Development of an instrument to measure collaboration and satisfaction about care decisions. *Journal of Advanced Nursing*, 20: 176–182.

Baggs, J. G. and Schmidt, M. (1988) Collaboration between nurse and physician. *Image Journal of Nursing Scholarship*, 20: 145–149.

Baggs, J. G. and Ryan, S. A. (1990) ICU nurse–physician collaboration and nursing satisfaction. *Nursing Economics*, 8: 386–392.

Baggs, J. G., Ryan, S., Phelps, C., Richeson, J. and Johnson, J. (1992) The association between interdisciplinary collaboration and patient outcomes. *Heart and Lung*, 21: 18–24.

Baggs, J. G., Schmidt, M. A., Mushlin, A. I., Eldredge, D. H., Oakes, D. and Hutson, A. D. (1997) Nurse–physician collaboration and satisfaction with the decision making process in three critical care units. *American Journal of Critical Care*, 6, 5: 393–399.

Baggs, J. G., Schmidt, M. H., Mushlin, A. I., Mitchell, P. H., Eldredge, D. H., Oakes D. and Hutson, A. D. (1999) Association between nurse–physician collaboration and patient outcomes in three intensive care units. *Critical Care Medicine*, 27, 9: 1991–1998.

Ball, C. (1997) Planning for the future: advanced nursing practice in critical care. *Intensive and Critical Care Nursing*, 13: 17–25.

Ball, C. (2001) *Legitimate Influence. The Key to Advanced Nursing Practice in Critical Care: A Grounded Theory Study.* Nursing Praxis, Chichester.

Barker, C. (1996) *The Health Care Policy Process.* Sage Publications, London.

Barriball, K. L. and While, A. (1994) Collecting data using a semi-structured interview: a discussion paper. *Journal of Advanced Nursing*, 19: 328–335.

Baruch, G. (1982) Moral tales: parents' stories of encounters with the health profession. Unpublished Ph.D. thesis, University of London.

Becker, H. S. (1958) Problems of inference and proof in participant observation. *American Sociological Review*, 23: 652–659.

Berg, B. L. (1989) *Qualitative Research Methods.* Allyn Bacon, Boston.

Benner, P. (1984) *From Novice to Expert: Excellence and Power in Clinical Nursing Practice.* Addison Wesley Publishing Company, Menlo Park, CA.

Blue, I. and Fitzgerald, M. (2002) Interprofessional relations: case studies of working relationships between registered nurses and general practitioners in rural Australia. *Journal of Clinical Nursing*, 11: 314–321.

Blumer, H. (1969) *Symbolic Interactionism: Perspective and Method*. Prentice Hall, New Jersey.

Bogdan, R. and Biklen, S. (1982) *Qualitative Research for Education: An Introduction to Theory and Methods*. Allyn Bacon, Boston.

Brilli, R. J., Speretz, A., Branson, R. D., Campbell, G. M., Cohen, H., Dasta, J. F., Harvey, M. A., Kelly, K. M., Rudis, M. I., Aude, A. C., Stone, J. R., Teres, D. and Weled, B. J. (2001) Critical care delivery in the ICU: defining clinical roles and the best practice model. *Critical Care Medicine* 29, 19: 2007–2019.

British Medical Association (1967) *Report of the Working Party on Intensive Care in the United Kingdom*. British Medical Association, London.

British Medical Association (2001) Workforce retention number one concern. October On-line: www.bma.org.uk

British Medical Association (2002) *The Future Healthcare Workforce: February 2002*. HPERU Discussion Paper 9. Retrieved from www.bma.org.uk/public/pols/

Brykcznski, K. A. (1989) An interpretive study describing the clinical judgement of nurse practitioners. *Scholarly Inquiry for Nursing Practice*, 3: 75–104.

Buchan, J. and Edwards, N. (2000) Nursing numbers in Britain: the argument for workforce planning. *British Medical Journal*, 320: 1067–1070.

Buckingham, C. and Adams, A. (2000) Classifying clinical decision making: interpreting nursing intuition, heuristics and medical diagnosis. *Journal of Advanced Nursing*, 32, 4: 990–998.

Burgess, R. G. (1984) *In the Field: An Introduction to Field Research*. George Allen and Unwin, London.

Burns, E. (1972) *Theatricality: A Study of Convention in the Theatre and in Social Life*. Longman, London.

Burr, G. (1996) Unfinished business: interviewing family members of critically ill patients. *Nursing Inquiry*, 3, 3: 172–177.

Busby, A. and Gilchrist, B. (1992) The role of the nurse in the medical ward round. *Journal of Advanced Nursing*, 17: 339–346.

Caines, E. (2001) Workforce retention number one concern. *Online BMA news*. Retrieved from www.bma.org.uk/nrczine.ns.../

Caines, K. (1996) Here to stay. *Nursing Standard*, 10, 45: 18.

Cannon, S. (1989) Social research in stressful settings: difficulties for the sociologist studying the treatment of breast cancer. *Sociology of Health and Illness*, 11, 1: 62–77.

Carper, B. A. (1978) Fundamental patterns of knowing in nursing. *Advances in Nursing Science*, 1, 1: 13–23.

Casteldine, G. (1991) The advanced nurse practitioner, Part 1. *Nursing Standard*, 5, 43: 34–36.

Casteldine, G. (1996) Clarifying and defining nursing role developments. *British Journal of Nursing*, 5, 21: 1338.

Chamberliss, D. (1996) *Beyond Caring: Hospitals, Nurses and the Social Organisation of Ethic*. University of Chicago Press, Chicago.

Chapman, C. (1976) The use of sociological theories and models in nursing. *Journal of Advanced Nursing*, 1, 2: 111–127.

Cheek, J. and Gibson, T. (1997) Policy matters: critical policy analysis and nursing. *Journal of Advanced Nursing*, 25: 668–672.

Chenitz, W. C. and Swanson, J. M. (1986) *From Practice to Grounded Theory: Qualitative Research in Nursing*. Addison-Wesley, Menlo Park, CA.

Cioffi, J. (2000) Nurses' experience of making decisions to call emergency assistance for their patients. *Journal of Advanced Nursing*, 32, 1: 108–114.

Coffey, A. (1999) *The Ethnographic Self. Fieldwork and the Representation of Identity*. Sage Publications, London.

Cohen, A. (1995) The market and professional frameworks. In *Interprofessional Issues in Community and Primary Health Care*. Owens, P., Carner, J., Foucher, J., eds. Macmillan, London.

Coluccio, M. and Maguire, P. (1983) Collaborative practice: becoming a reality through primary nursing. *Nursing Administration Quarterly*, 7: 59–63.

Cott, C. (1997) 'We decide, you carry it out': a social network analysis of multi-disciplinary long term care teams. *Social Science Medicine*, 45, 9: 1411–1421.

Cray, L. (1989) A collaborative project: initiating a family intervention program in a medical intensive care unit. *Focus on Critical Care*, 16, 3: 213–218.

Crosby, D. L. and Rees, G. A. D. (1994) Provision of post-operative care in UK hospitals. *Annals of the Royal College of Surgeons in England*, 75: 14–18.

Crow, R. A., Chase, J. and Lamond, D. (1995) The cognitive component of nursing assessment: an analysis. *Journal of Advanced Nursing*, 22: 206–212.

Curry, S. (1995) Identifying family needs and stresses in the intensive care unit. *British Journal of Nursing*, 12: 4–10.

Daily Telegraph (2000) Flu outbreak leaves only 11 beds for intensive care in London. *Daily Telegraph*, 6 Jan.

Darvas, J. A. and Hawkins, L. G. (2002) What makes a good intensive care unit: a nursing perspective. *Australian Critical Care*, 15, 2: 77–82.

Davies, C. (1995) *Gender and the Professional Predicament of Nursing*. Open University Press, Buckingham.

Davies, C. (1996) A new vision of professionalism. *Nursing Times*, 92, 46: 54–56.

Davies, C., Salvage, J. and Smith, R. (1999) Doctors and nurses: changing family values? *British Medical Journal*, 319: 463–464.

Davis, D. L. (1992) The meaning of menopause in a Newfoundland fishing village. *In Qualitative Research Methods*. Morse, J. M., ed. Sage, Newbury Park, CA.

Day, H. W. (1963) An intensive coronary area. *Diseases of the Chest*, 44: 423–425.

DeAngelis, C. (1994) Nurse practitioner redux. *Journal of American Medical Association*, 271, 11: 868–871.

Delamont, S. and Atkinson, P. (1995) *Fighting Familiarity*. Hampton Creskill, New Jersey.

Denyes, M. J., O'Connor, N. A., Oakley, D. and Ferguson, S. (1998). Integrating nursing theory, practice and research through collaborative research. *Journal of Advanced Nursing* 14 (2) 141–145.

Denzin, N. K. (1970) *The Research Act in Society*. Butterworth, London.

Denzin, N. K. (1992) *Symbolic Interactionism and Cultural Studies: The Politics of Interpretation*. Blackwell Publishers, Massachusetts.

Department of Health (1989) *Working for Patients*. Cm 555 HMSO, London.

Department of Health (1990) *The National Health Service and Community Care Act*. HMSO, London.

Department of Health (1991) *Junior Doctors: The New Deal*. National Health Service Medical Executive, London.

Department of Health (1992) *The Health of the Nation: A Strategy for Health in England*. HMSO, London.

Department of Health (1993) *Vision for the Future*. National Health Service Medical Executive, London.

Department of Health (1996a) *Guidelines on Admission to and Discharge from Intensive Care and High Dependency Units*. Department of Health, London.

Department of Health (1996b) *The New National Health Service: A Service with Ambitions*. Cm 3425, HMSO, London.

Department of Health (1997) *Primary Care: Delivering for the Future*. HMSO, London.

Department of Health (1998) *A First Class Service. Quality in the New NHS*. Department of Health, London.

Department of Health (1999) *Making a Difference: Strengthening the Nursing, Midwives and Health Visitors' Contribution to Health and Health Care*. Department of Health, London.

Department of Health (2000a) *Comprehensive Critical Care: A Review of Adult Critical Care Services*. Department of Health, London.

Department of Health (2000b) *The NHS Plan: A Plan for Investment, a Plan for Reform*. Department of Health, London.

Department of Health (2001a) *The Nursing Contribution to the Provision of Comprehensive Critical Care Services for Adults: A Strategic Action Plan*. Department of Health, London.

Department of Health (2001b) *Shifting the Balance of Power: The Next Steps*. Department of Health, London.

Department of Health (2002) *Unfinished Business. Proposals for Reforms of the Senior House Officer Grade. A Report by Sir Liam Donaldson Chief Medical Officer for England. A Paper Consultation*. Department of Health, London.

Department of Health (2003) *Keeping the NHS Local: A New Direction of Travel*. Department of Health, London.

Department of Health and Social Security (1972) *Report of the Committee on Nursing*. HMSO, London.

Dillon, A. and George, S. (1997) Advanced neonatal practitioners in the United Kingdom: where are they and what do they do? *Journal of Advanced Nursing*, 25: 257–264.

Dimond, B. (1995) When the nurse wields the scalpel. *British Journal of Nursing*, 4, 2: 65–66.

Dingwall, R. (1980) Ethics and ethnography. *Sociological Review*, 28, 4: 871–891.

Dorman, S. (1996) Contracting for intensive care services. *Nursing in Critical Care*, 1, 1: 13–16.

Dowling, S. and Barrett, S. (1991) *Doctors in the Making: The Experiences of the Pre-registration Year*. University of Bristol, Bristol.

Dragsted, L. and Qvist, J. (1992) Epidemiology of intensive care in UK hospitals. *International Journal of Technological Assessment in Health Care*, 8: 395–407.

Dunbar, S. and Bryan-Brown, C. (1988) Collaborative practice model. In *International Conference on Collaborative Practice*. American Association of Critical Care Nurses, Newport Beach.

Durkheim, E. (1933) *The Division of Labour in Society*. Colliere-Macmillan, London.

Edbrookes, D. (1996) High dependency – so much promise – so little progress. *Care of the Critically Ill*, 12, 3: 80–81.

Edbrookes, D. L., Stevens, V. G., Hibbert, C. L., Mann, A. J. and Wilson, A. J. (1997) A new method of accurately identifying costs of individual patients in intensive care: the initial results. *Intensive Care Medicine*, 23: 645–650.

Ekman, I. and Segestein, K. (1995) Deputed power of medical control: the hidden message in the ritual of oral shift reports. *Journal of Advanced Nursing*, 22: 1006–1011.

Elliot, P. A. (1995) The development of advanced practice: 1, *British Journal of Nursing*, 4, 11: 633–636.

Elston, M. A. (1991) The politics of professional power – medicine in a changing health service. In *The Sociology of the Health Services*, Gabe, J., Calnan, M. and Bury, M., eds. Routledge, London.

Ely, M., Vinz, R., Downing, M. and Anzul, M. (1997) *On Writing Qualitative Research: Living by Words*. Falmer, London.

Endacott, R. (1996) Staffing intensive care units: a consideration of contemporary issues. *Intensive and Critical Care Nursing*, 12: 193–199.

Fagin, C. M. (1992) Collaboration between nurses and physicians: no longer a choice. *Academic Medicine*, 67: 295–303.

Fairman, J. (1992) Watchful vigilance: nursing care, technology and the development of intensive care units. *Nursing Research*, 41, 1: 56–59.

Fantus, B. (1937) Therapy of County Cook Hospital: blood preservation. *Journal of American Medical Association*, 109: 128.

Fatchett, A. (1996) A chance for community nurses to shape the agenda. *Nursing Times*, 92, 45: 40–42.

Fatchett, A. (1998) *Nursing in the New National Health Service: Modern, Dependable*. Balliere Tindall, Edinburgh.

Fitzgerald, L. (1994) Moving clinicians into management: a professional challenge or threat? *Journal of Management in Medicine*, 8, 6: 32–44.

Fitzgerald, L., Duffour, Y. (1997) Clinical management as boundary management: a comparative analysis of Canadian and United Kingdom health care institutions. *International Journal of Public Sector Management*, 10, 1/2: 5–20.

Flynn, R. (1992) *Structures of Control in Health Management*. Routledge, London.

Fonteyn, M. E. (1999) *Thinking Strategies for Nursing Practice*. Lippincott, New York.

Foucault, M. (1975) *The Birth of the Clinic: An Archaeology of Medical Perception*. Vintage Books, New York.

Fowler, M. D. M. (1989) Moral distress and the shortage of critical care nurses. *Heart and Lung*, 18, 3: 314–315.

Fox, N. J. (1993) Discourse, organisation and the surgical ward round. *Sociology of Health and Illness*, 15: 16–42.

Freidson, E. (1970) *The Profession of Medicine: A Study of the Sociology of Applied Knowledge*. University of Chicago Press, Chicago.

Freidson, E. (1976) The division of labour as social interaction. *Sociological Problems*, 23: 304–313.

Freidson, E. (1994) *Professionalism Reborn*. Polity Press, Cambridge.

Frost, S. (1996) Perspectives on advanced practice: an educationalist's view. In *Advanced Nursing Practice*. Rolfe, G. and Fulbrook, P. eds. ButterworthHeinemann, Oxford.

Gable, J., Kellener, D. and Williams, G. (1994) *Challenging Medicine*. Routledge, London.

Gadow, S. (1985) Nurse and patient: the caring relationship. In *Caring, Curing, Coping*. Bishop, A. H. and Scudder, J. R. eds. University of Alabama Press, Tuscaloosa.

Gallagher, A. (1995) Medical and nursing ethics: never the twain? *Nursing Ethics*, 2, 2: 95–101.

Gamarnikow, E. (1978) Sexual division of labour: the case in nursing. In *Feminism and Materialism*, Kuhn, A. and Holpe, E., eds. Routledge and Kegan Paul, London.

Gamarnikow, E. (1991) Nurse or woman: gender and professionalism in reformed nursing 1860–1923. In *Anthropology and Nursing*. Holden, P. and Littleworth, J., eds. Routledge, London.

Geer, B. (1964) First days in the field. In *Sociologists at Work*. Hammond, P. E., ed. Basic Books, New York.

Geertz, C. (1973) *The Interpretation of Culture*. Basic Books, New York.

Geertz, C. (1988) *Working and Lives: The Anthropologist as Author*. Stanford University Press, Stanford.

General Medical Council (1995) *Good Medical Practice Guidance from the General Medical Council*. General Medical Council, London.

Gerrish, K. (1997) Being a marginal native: dilemmas of the participant observer. *Nurse Researcher*, 5, 1: 26–34.

Gilligan, C. (1982) *In a Different Voice*. Harvard University Press, Cambridge.

Gillon, R. (1992) Caring, men and women, nurses and doctors and health care ethics. *Journal of Medical Ethics*, 18: 171–182.

Glaser, B. G. and Strauss, A. L. (1967) *The Discovery of Grounded Theory*. Aldine De Gruyter, New York.

Goffman, E. (1959) *The Presentation of Self in Everyday Life*. Penguin, Harmondsworth.

Gold, R. (1958) Roles in sociological field observation. *Social Forces*, 36, 3: 217–223.

Goldacre, M. (1998) Planning the United Kingdom's medical workforce. *British Medical Journal*, 3, 16: 1846–1847.

Green, J. and Armstrong, D. (1993) Achieving rational management: bed managers and the crisis in emergency admissions. *The Sociological Review*, 43: 743–764.

Grimley, J. (1986) Critical educational policy analysis. A discussion of perspectives. *Australian Journal of Teacher Education*, 11, 2: 19–25.

Grundstein-Amado, R. (1992) Differences in ethical decision making processes among nurses and doctors. *Journal of Advanced Nursing*, 17: 129–137.

Halford, S., Savage, M. and Witz, A. (1997) *Gender, Careers and Organisations. Current Developments in Banking, Nursing and Local Government*. Macmillan, Basingstoke.

Hall, P., Land, H., Parker, R. and Webb, A. (1975) *Change, Choice and Conflict in Social Policy*. Heinemann, London.

Ham, C. and Hill, M. (1986) *The Policy Process in the Modern Capitalist State*. Wheatsheaf Books, Brighton.

Ham, C. (1992) *Health Policy in Britain*. 3rd edn. Macmillan, Basingstoke.

Hammersley, M. (1993) *Social Research: Philosophy, Politics and Practice*. Sage, London.

Hammersley, M. and Atkinson, P. (1983) *Ethnography: Principles in Practice*, Tavistock, London.

Hammersley, M. and Atkinson, P. (1995) *Ethnography: Principles in Practice*. 2nd edn. Routledge, London.

Hamric, B. and Spross, J. (1989) *The Clinical Nurse Specialist in Theory and Practice*. Saunders, London.

Hancock C. (1995) *Care in the Year 2000: In Nursing Beyond Tradition and Conflict.* Jolley, M. and Brykczynska, G., ed. Mosby, London.

Harrison, S. and Pollitt, C. (1994) *Controlling Health Professionals: The Future of Work and Organisations in the National Health Service.* Open University Press, Buckingham.

Harrison, A. and Bruscini, S. (1995) *Health Care in the UK 1994/5.* Kings Fund Policy Institute, London.

Harrison, S., Hunter, D. J., Marnoch, G. and Pollitt, C. (1992) *Just Managing: Power and Culture in the National Health Service.* Macmillan, Basingstoke.

Harwood, A. and Boufford, J. (1993) *Managing Clinical Services: A Consensus Statement of Principles of Effective Clinical Management.* British Association of Medical Managers, London.

Hatt, G. (1998) Uncertainty in medical decision making. *In Health Matters: A Sociology of Illness, Prevention and Care.* Peterson, A. and Waddell, C., eds. Open University Press, Buckingham.

Hayes, E. (1990) Needs of family members of critically ill patients: a Northern Ireland perspective. *Intensive and Critical Care Nursing,* 6: 23–29.

Helman, C. G. (1990) *Culture, Health and Illness.* ButterworthHeinemann.

Henderson, V. A. (1980) Preserving the essence of nursing in a technological age. *Journal of Advanced Nursing,* 5: 245–260.

Henneman, E. (1995) Collaboration: a concept analysis. *Journal of Advanced Nursing,* 21: 103–109.

Henneman, E., Dracup, K., Ganz, T., Molnyenne, O. and Cooper, C. (2001) Effect of a collaborative weaning plan on patient outcome in a critical care setting. *Critical Care Medicine,* 29, 2: 297–303.

Hennessy, D. and Spurgeon, P. (2000) *Health Policy and Nursing: Influence, Development and Impact.* Macmillan, Basingstoke.

HM Treasury (2002) *Securing Our Future Health: Taking a Long-term View* (Wanless Report). HM Treasury, London.

Hickey, J. V., Ouimette, R. M. and Venegoni, I. (1996) *Advanced Practice Nursing.* Lippincott, PA.

Higgs, J. and Jones, M. (1995) *Clinical Reasoning in the Heath Professions.* Butterworth-Heinemann, Oxford.

Hilderley, L. (1991) Nurse–physician collaborative practice: the clinical nurse specialist in a radiation oncology practice. *Oncology Nursing Forum,* 18: 585–591.

Hochschild, A. R. (1983) *The Managed Heart: Commercialisation of Human Feeling.* University of California Press, Berkeley, CA.

Hogwood, B. and Gunn, L. (1984) *Policy Analysis for the Real World.* Oxford University Press, Oxford.

Holloway, I. and Wheeler, S. (1996) *Qualitative Research for Nurses.* Blackwell Science, Oxford.

Hughes, D. (1988) When a nurse knows best: some aspects of doctor/nurse interaction in a casualty department. *Sociology of Health and Illness,* 10: 1–22.

Hughes, E. C. (1984) *The Sociological Eye.* Transaction Books, London.

Hugman, R. (1991) *Power in the Caring Professions.* Macmillan, Basingstoke.

Humphrey, L. (1970) *Tearoom Trade.* Aldine, Chicago.

Hunt, G. and Wainwright, P. (1994) *Expanding the Role of the Nurse: The Scope of Professional Practice.* Blackwell Scientific, Oxford.

Illich, I. (1977) *The Limits to Medicine.* Penguin, London.

Intensive Care Society (1990) *Standards for Intensive Care Units*. Intensive Care Society, London.

IPPR (Institute for Public Policy Research) (2002) *Rethinking Professionalism: The First Step for Patient-focussed Care?* By Salvage, J. Retrieved from http//ippr.org/research/index.php?project=13&current=24

Jacques, R. (1993) Untheorized dimensions of caring work: caring as a structural practice and caring as a way of seeing. *Nursing Administration Quarterly*, 17, 2: 1–10.

James, N. (1989) Emotional labour: skills and work in the social regulation of feelings. *Sociological Review*, 37: 15–42.

Johnson, J. M. (1975) *Doing Field Research*. Free Press, New York.

Jolley, M. and Brykczyskia, G. (1993) A sociologist's view: the handmaiden's theory. In *Nursing Its Hidden Agendas*. Jolley, M. and Brykczyskia, G., eds. Edward Arnold, London.

Jones, C. (1987) Handmaiden mentality. *Nursing Times*, 83, 40: 59.

Jones, L. J. (1994) *The Social Context of Health and Health Work*. Macmillan, Basingstoke.

Jowett, N. (1986) The junior doctor on the intensive care unit. *Intensive and Critical Care Nursing*, 1: 177–179.

Kalisch, B. J. and Kalisch, P. A. (1977) An analysis of the sources of physician–nurse conflict. *Journal of Nursing Administration*, 7: 51–57.

Kassirer, J. P. and Gorry, G. A. (1978) Clinical problem solving: a behavioural analysis. *Annals of Internal Medicine*, 89: 245–255.

Keen, J. and Malby, R. (1992) Nursing power and practice in the United Kingdom National Health Service. *Journal of Advanced Nursing*, 17: 863–870.

King, M. B. (1990) Clinical nurse specialist collaboration with physicians. *Clinical Nurse Specialist*, 4: 172–177.

Klein, R. (1983) *The Politics of the National Health Service*. Longman, London.

Knaus, W. A. (1980) *Collaboration in Organisations*. Human Science Press, New York.

Knaus, W. A., Draper, E. A., Wagner, D. P. and Zimmerman, J. E. (1986) An evaluation of outcome from intensive care in major medical centres. *Annals of Internal Medicine*, 104: 410–418.

Koerner, B. L., Cohen, J. R. and Armstrong, D. M. (1985) Collaborative practice and patient satisfaction: impact and selected outcomes. *Evaluation of the Health Professions*, 8: 299–321.

Kolff, W. J. (1947) *New Ways of Treating Uraemia*. Churchill Livingstone, London.

Krueger, R. A. (1994) *Focus Groups: A Practical Guide for Applied Research*. Sage Publications, Thousand Oaks, CA.

Lamb, G. S. and Napadano, R. J. (1984) Physician–nurse practitioner interaction patterns in primary care practices. *American Journal of Public Health*, 74: 26–29.

Lassen, H. C. A. (1953) A preliminary report of the 1952 epidemic of poliomyelitis in Copenhagen with special reference to the treatment of acute respiratory insufficiency. *The Lancet*, 1: 37–41.

Lathlean, J. (1996a) The challenges of longitudinal ethnographic research in nursing. *Nursing Times Research*, 1, 1: 38–43.

Lathlean, J. (1996b) Ethical issues for nursing research: a methodological focus. *Nursing Times Research*, 1, 3: 175–183.

Lawler, J. (1997) *The Body in Nursing*. Churchill Livingstone, Melbourne.

Layder, D. (1998) The reality of social domains: implications for theory and method.

In *Knowing the Social World*. May, T. and Williams, M., eds. Open University Press, Buckingham.

Leathard, A. (1994) *Going Interprofessional: Working Together for Health and Welfare*. Routledge, London.

Leatt, P. and Schneck, R. (1981) Nursing and technology: a replication. *Administrative Science Quarterly*, 26: 225–226.

LeCompte, M. D. and Goetz, J. P. (1982) Problems of reliability and validity in ethnographic research. *Review of Educational Research*, 52, 1: 31–60.

Lee, R. (1993) *Doing Research on Sensitive Topics*. Sage Publications, London.

Leininger, M. (1985) *Qualitative Research Methods in Nursing*. Grune Stratton, New York.

Levitt, R. and Wall, A. (1992) *The Re-organised National Health Service*. Chapman and Hall, London.

Liaschenko, J. (1998) The shift from the closed to the open body: ramifications for nursing testimony. In *Philosophical Issues in Nursing*. Edwards, S. D., ed. Macmillan, Basingstoke.

Light, D. (1993) Countervailing powers: the changing character of the medical profession in the United States. In *The Changing Character of the Medical Profession*. Hafferty, F. and McKinley, J. B., eds. Oxford University Press, Oxford.

Lilford, R. J., Parker, S. G., Braunholtz, D. A. and Chard, J. (1998) Decision analysis and the implementation of research findings. *British Medical Journal*, 317: 405–409.

Lincoln, Y. S. and Guba, E. G. (1994) *Naturalistic Enquiry*. Sage, Newbury Park, CA.

Lofland, J. and Lofland, L. H. (1995) *Analysing Social Settings: A Guide to Qualitative Observation and Analysis*. 3rd edn. Wadsworth, Belmont, CA.

Macara, S. (1996) Reforms have led the National Health staff to despair. *British Medical Journal News Review*, April: 35.

Mackay, L. (1989) *Nursing a Problem*. Open University Press, Buckingham.

Macleod-Clarke, J. (1983) Nurse–patient communication in surgical wards. In *Nursing Research: Ten Studies in Patient Care*. Wilson Barnett, J., ed. Wiley, Chichester.

Mahon, J. (1995) *A National Health Service? The Restructuring of Health Care in Britain since 1979*. Macmillan, Basingstoke.

Makaram, S. (1995) Interprofessional co-operation. *Medical Education*, 29, supplement 1: 65–69.

Malinowski, B. (1922) *Argonauts of the Western Pacific*. Routledge, London.

Manias, E. and Street, A. (2001a) The interplay of knowledge and dominance between nurses and doctors in critical care. *International Journal of Nursing Studies*, 38: 129–140.

Manias, E. and Street, A. (2001b) Nurse–doctor interactions during critical care ward rounds. *Journal of Clinical Nursing*, 10: 442–450.

Manley, K. (1990) The birth of a nursing development unit. *Nursing Standard*, 21, 4: 36–38.

Manley, K. (1996) Advanced practice is not about medicalising nursing roles. *Nursing in Critical Care*, 1, 2: 56–57.

Mann, R. E. (1992) Preserving humanity in an age of technology. *Intensive and Critical Care Nursing*, 8: 54–59.

Manning, P. (1992) *Erving Goffman and Modern Sociology*. Polity Press, Cambridge.

Mark, A. L. and Dopson, S. (1999) *Organisational Behaviour in Health Care: The Research Agenda*. Macmillan Business, Basingstoke.

Marnoch, G. (1996) *Doctors and Management in the National Health Service*. Open University Press, Basingstoke.

Marnoch, G. and Ross, K. (1998) *Flags and Badges: Legitimacy in the New National Health Service*. Working Paper, Department of Management Studies, University of Aberdeen.

Masterson, A. (1994) Making and Implementing Social Policy. In *Nursing and Social policy: Care in Context*. Gough, P. Maslin-Prothero, S. and Masterson, A., eds. ButterworthHeinemann, London.

Masterson, A. (2002) Cross-boundary working: a macro-political analysis of the impact on professional roles. *Journal of Clinical Nursing*, 11: 331–339.

Mather, H. (2001) *The RCP Specialist Registrar Shift Survey. April. On Behalf of the RCP Trainees' Committee*. Retrieved from hmarthur@onetel.netuk

May, T. (1993) Documentary research. In *Social Research, Issues, Methods and Process*. Open University Press, Buckingham.

McCallin, A. (2001) Interdisciplinary practice – a matter of teamwork: an integrated literature review. *Journal of Clinical Nursing*, 10: 419–428.

McGee, P., Casteldine, G. and Brown, R. (1996) A survey of specialist and advanced nursing practice in England. *British Journal of Specialist Nursing*, 5: 682–686.

McKee, L., Marnoch, G. and Dinnie, N. (1999) Medical managers: puppetmasters or puppets? Sources of power and influence in clinical directorates. In *Organisational Behaviour in Health Care: The Research Agenda*. Mark, A. L. and Dopson, M., eds. Macmillan Business, Basingstoke.

McKee, M. and Clarke, A. (1995) Guidelines, enthusiasms, uncertainty, and the limits to purchasing. *British Medical Journal*, 310: 101–104.

McKeown, T. (1976) *The Modern Rise of Population*. Arnold, London.

Mechanic, D. (1991) Sources of countervailing power in medicine. *Journal of Health Politics, Policy and Law*, 16, 3: 485–506.

Medical Workforce Standing Advisory Committee (1997) *Planning the Workforce: The Third Report*. Department of Health, London.

Merrell, J. and Williams, A. (1994) Participant observation and informed consent: relationships and tactical decision making in nursing research. *Nursing Ethics*, 1, 3: 163–172.

Miccolo, M. A. and Spanier, A. H. (1993) Critical care management in the 1990s. Making collaborative practice work. *Critical Care Clinics*, 9, 3: 443–453.

Miles, M. B. and Huberman, A. M. (1994) *Qualitative Data Analysis*, 2nd edn. Sage Publications, Thousand Oaks, CA.

Mills, C. (1997) The consultant nurse: a model for advanced practice. *Nursing Times*, 92, 33: 36–37.

Minh-Ha, T. T. (1991) *When the Moon Waxes Red*. Routledge, New York.

Miranda, D. R., Moreno, R. and Lapichino, G. (1997) Nine equivalents of nursing manpower use scores (NEMS) *Intensive Care Medicine*, 23: 760–765.

Mitchell, C. (1983) Case and situational analysis. *Sociological Review*, 31, 2: 187–211.

Moore, G. T. (1990) Doctors as managers: frustrating tensions. In *The Future of Acute Services: Doctors as Managers*. Costain, D., ed. Kings Fund Centre, London.

Moser, C. and Kalton, G. (1983) *Survey Methods in Social Investigations*. Heinemann, London.

National Health Service Executive (1983) *Enquiry into NHS management* (The Griffiths Report). NHSE London.

National Health Service Executive (1999) *Clinical Governance: Quality in the New N.H.S. Executive Summary*, NHSE Leeds.

Netherton, S. (1995) *The Sociology of Health and Illness*. Polity Press, Cambridge.

Neubauer, J. F. (1993) Redesign: managing role changes and building new teams. *Seminar for Nurse Managers*, 1, 1: 26–32.

Newman, J. and Clarke, J. (1994) Going about our business? The managerialisation of public services. In *Managing Social Policy*. Clarke, J. and McLaughlin E., eds. Sage, London.

Nightingale, F. (1863) *Notes on Hospitals*. Longmans, Green, London.

Noc, M. and Weil, M. H. (1996) Critical care today. In *Critical Care Standards Audit and Ethics*. Tinker, J., Browne, D. and Sibbald, W. J., eds. Arnold Press, New York.

Norheim, C. (1989) Family needs of patients having coronary artery bypass graft surgery during the intra-operative period. *Heart and Lung*, 18: 622–626.

Norrie, P. (1997) Ethical decision making in intensive care: are nurses suitable patient advocates? *Intensive and Critical Care Nursing*, 13, 3: 167–169.

O'Hanlon, M. and Gibbon, S. (1996) Advanced practice. *Nursing Management*, 2, 10: 12–13.

Oberle, K. and Hughes, D. (2001) Doctors' and nurses' perceptions of ethical problems in end of life decisions. *Journal of Advanced Nursing*, 33, 6: 707–715.

Oh, T. E. (1996) The development, utilisation and cost implications of intensive care medicine: strategies for the future. In *Critical Care Standards Audit and Ethics*. Tinker, J., Browne, D., Sibbald, W. J., eds. Arnold Press, New York.

Ovretveit, J., Mathias, P. and Thompson, T. (1997) *Interprofessional Working for Health and Social Care*. Macmillan, Basingstoke.

Owens, P. and Glennerster, H. (1990) *Nursing in Conflict*. Macmillan, London.

Oxford English Dictionary (1990) *The Concise Oxford Dictionary of Current English*. 8th edn. Clarendon Press, Oxford.

Packwood, T., Keen, J. and Buxton, M. (1991) *Hospitals in Transition: The Resource Management Experience*. Open University Press. Milton Keynes.

Paniagua, H. (1995) The scope of advanced nursing: action potential for practice nurses. *British Journal of Nursing*, 4, 5: 269–274.

Parish, C. (2003) Another door opens. *Nursing Standard*, 17, 19: 12–13.

Parker, J. and Gardner, G. (1992) The silence and the silencing of the nurses voice: a reading of patient progress notes. *Australian Journal of Advanced Nursing*, 9, 2: 3–9.

Parker, J. and Wiltshire, J. (1995) The handover: three modes of nursing practice knowledge. In *Scholarship in the Discipline of Nursing*. Gray, G. and Pratt, R., eds. Churchill Livingstone, Edinburgh.

Payne, D. (1999) Nice work if you can get it. *Nursing Times*, 95, 29: 12.

Pearson, A. (1983) *The Clinical Nursing Unit*. Heinemann, London.

Phillips, S. (1996) Labouring the emotions: expanding the remit of nursing work? *Journal of Advanced Nursing*, 24, 1: 139–143.

Pickles, A. (1999) Nurse versus technician: the dilemma of intensive care nursing. *Nursing in Critical Care*, 4, 3: 148–150.

Pilcher, T., Odell, M., Bray, K., Clarke, S., Gardiner, J., Orr, R. and Stirton, H. (2001) Nurse–patient ratios in critical care. *Nursing in Critical Care*, 6: 59–63.

Pilliteri, A. and Ackerman, M. (1993) The doctor nurse game: a comparison of 100 years. *Nursing Outlook*, 41: 113–116.

Plummer, K. (1990) Herbert Blumer and the life history tradition. *Symbolic Interaction*, 13, 2: 125–144.

Porter, S. (1991) A participant observation study of power relations between nurses and doctors in a general hospital. *Journal of Advanced Nursing*, 16: 728–735.

Porter, S. (1993) Critical realist ethnography: the case of racism and professionalism in a medical setting. *Sociology*, 27: 591–609.

Porter, S. (1995) *Nursing's Relationship with Medicine: A Critical Realist Ethnography*. Developments in nursing and health care. Avebury, Basingstoke.

Porter, S. (1996) Contra-Focault: nurses, soldiers and power. *Sociology*, 30, 1: 59–78.

Porter, S. (1998) *Social Theory and Nursing Practice*. Macmillan, Basingstoke.

Prescott, P. A. and Bowen, S. A. (1985) Physician–nurse relationship. *Annals of Internal Medicine*, 103: 127–133.

Pringle, R. (1989) *Secretaries Talk: Sexuality, Power and Work*. Verso, London.

Pursey, A. and Brocklehurst, N. (1996) Developing the nursing contribution to purchasing. Unpublished report. West Midlands Regional Health Authority.

Rafferty, A. M. (1992) Nursing policy and the nationalisation of nursing: the representation of crisis and the crisis of representation In *Policy Issues in Nursing*. Robinson, J., Gray, A. and Elkan, R. eds. Open University Press, Milton Keynes.

Ranade, W. (1994) *A Future for the NHS? Health Care in the 1990's*. Longman, London.

Redfern, S. (1997) Reactions to nurses' expanding practice. *Nursing Times*, 93, 32: 45–47.

Reeve, T. (1993) Coherent and consistent quality assurance and utilisation review activities. In *Public and Private Hospitals in Australia: Casemix Development Programme*. Canberra, Australia.

Reid, B. (1991) Developing and documenting a qualitative methodology, *Journal of Advanced Nursing*, 16: 544–551.

Reid, S. (1998) Nursing and new roles. In *Advanced Nursing Practice*. Rolfe, G. and Fulbrook, P., eds. ButterworthHeinemann, Oxford.

Rennie, M. (1999) The facts. *British Journal of Intensive Care*, Jan./Feb.: 5.

Roberts, S. L. (1987) The role of collaborative diagnosis in critical care. *Critical Care Nurse*, 7: 81–86.

Robertson, D. W. (1996) Ethical theory, ethnography and differences between doctors and nurses in approaches to patient care. *Journal of Medical Education*, 22: 292–299.

Robinson, J. (1997) Power, politics and policy analysis in nursing. In *Nursing: A Knowledge Base for practice* 2nd edn. Perry, A. and Jolley, M., eds. Arnold, London.

Robinson, J. and Strong, P. (1987) *Professional Nursing Advice after Griffiths: An Interim Report*. Nursing Policy Studies 1. Coventry: Nursing Policy Studies Centre, University of Warwick.

Robinson, J., Strong, P. and Elkan, R. (1989) *Griffiths and the Nurses: A National Survey of CNAs*. Nursing policy Studies 4. Coventry: Nursing Policy Studies Centre, University of Warwick.

Robinson, J., Gray, A. and Elkan, R. (1993) *Policy Issues in Nursing*. Open University Press, Milton Keynes.

Robotham, M. (1999) What do you think of doctors? *Nursing Times*, 95, 2: 24–27.

Ross, F. and Mackenzie, A. (1996) *Nursing in Primary Health Care: Policy into Practice*. Routledge, London.

Roth, M. D. and Daze, A.-M. (1984) Are nurses practising medicine in the intensive care unit? *Dimensions of Critical Care Nursing*, 3, 4: 230–237.

Royal College of Nursing (1992) *The Value of Nursing.* Royal College of Nursing, London.

Royal College of Nursing Critical Care Forum (1997) *The Nature of Nursing Work in Intensive Care: Results of a Telephone Survey.* Royal College of Nursing, London.

Royal College of Nursing (1998) *The New Primary Care Groups: The Knowledge and Skills Nurses Need to Make Them a Real Success.* Royal College of Nursing, London.

Royal College of Physicians (2001) Two years on: workload heavy, doctor shortage still acute. Retrieved from www.rcplondon.ac.uk/news/news.asp.Pr, 19 Feb. 2002.

Royal College of Physicians (2002) Physician's job satisfaction reaches new low. Retrieved from www.rcplondon.ac.uk/news/news. Feb. 2002.

Rubel, T. L. and Thomas, K. (1976) Support for a 2 fold dimensional model of conflict behaviour. *Organisational Behaviour and Human Performance*, 16: 145.

Rudge, T. (1996) (Re)writing ethnography: the unsettling questions for nursing research raised by post structural approaches to the field. *Nursing Inquiry*, 3: 140–152.

Saks, M. (1990) Does it pay to care? In *Circles of Care: Work and Identity in Women's Lives.* Abel, E. K., Nelson, M. K., eds. SUNY Press, New York.

Salvage, J. (1988) Professionalism or a struggle for survival? A consideration of current proposals for the reform of nursing in the United Kingdom. *Journal of Advanced Nursing*, 13: 515–519.

Salvage, J. and Smith, R. (2000) Doctors and nurses: doing it differently: the time is ripe for a major reconstruction. *British Medical Journal*, 320, 7241: 1019–1020.

Sandelowski, M., Holditch-Davis, D. and Harris, B. G. (1992) Using qualitative and quantitative methods in the transition to parenthood of infertile couples. In *Qualitative Methods in Family Research.* Gilgun, J. F., Daly, K. and Handel, G. eds. Sage, Newbury Park, CA.

Schneider, R. (1997) The effects on nurses of treatment withdrawal decisions made in ICUs and SCBUs. *Nursing in Critical Care*, 2, 4: 174–185.

Scholes, J. (1998) Therapeutic use of self: a component of advanced nursing practice. In *Advanced Nursing Practice.* Rolfe, G. and Fulbrook, P., eds. Butterworth-Heinemann, Oxford.

Seymour, J. E. (2001) *Critical Moments. Death and Dying in Intensive Care.* Open University Press, Buckingham.

Shilling, R. J. and Stoller, D. L. (1993) Opening the door to collaboration with physicians. Unpublished manuscript. Cited in *Advanced Practice Nursing: A Guide to Professional Development.* Snyder, M. and Mico, M. eds. Springer, New York.

Silverman, D. (1993) *Interpreting Qualitative Data: Methods for Analysing Talk, Text and Interaction.* Sage Publications, London.

Sinclair, S. (1997) *Making Doctors. An Institutional Apprenticeship.* Berg, Oxford.

Smart, C. (1984) *The Ties That Bind: Law, Marriage and the Reproduction of Patriarchal Relationships.* Routledge & Kegan Paul, London.

Smith, B. G. (1998a) Training in intensive care medicine. *Care of the Critically Ill*, 14, 2: 71–75.

Smith, M. (1998b) Who should run intensive care units? *Care of the Critically Ill*, 14, 4: 113–115.

Soderberg, A., Gilje, F. and Norberg, A. (1997) Dignity in situations of ethical difficulty in intensive care. *Intensive and Critical Care Nursing*, 13, 3: 135–144.

Sorrells-Jones, J. (1997) The challenge of making it real: interdisciplinary practice in a seamless organisation. *Nursing Administration Quarterly*, 21, 2: 20–30.

Spatz, D. L. (1996) The role of advanced practice nurses in the 21st century. *Nursing Clinics of North America*, 31, 2: 269–277.

Spradley, J. P. (1979) *The Ethnographic Interview*. Harcourt Brace Janovich, Fort Worth.

Spradley, J. P. (1980) *Participant Observation*. Holt, Rhinehart and Winston, New York.

Spurgeon, P. (2000) Implications of policy development for the nursing profession. In *Health Policy and Nursing Influence, Development and Impact*. Hennessy, D. and Spurgeon, P. eds. Macmillan, Basingstoke.

Stacey, M. (1991) Medical sociology and health policy: an historical overview. In *The Sociology of the Health Service*. Gabe, J., Calnan, M. and Bury, M., eds. Routledge, London.

Stanley, L. and Wise, S. (1983) *Breaking Out: Feminist Consciousness and Feminist Research*. Routledge & Kegan Paul, London.

Steel, J. (1986) *Issues in Collaborative Practice*. Grune Stratton, Boston.

Steier, F. (1995) *Research and Reflexivity*. Sage Publications, London.

Stein, L. (1967) The doctor nurse game. *Archives of General Psychiatry*, 16: 699–703.

Stein, L. I., Watts, D. T. and Howell, T. (1990) The doctor nurse game revisited. *Nursing Outlook*, Nov./Dec.: 264–268.

Stephenson, J. and Greer, L. (1981) Ethnographers in their own cultures: two Appalachian cases. *Human Organisation*, 40, 2: 123–130.

Stichler, J. F. (1995) Professional interdependence: the art of collaboration. *Advanced Practice Nursing Quarterly*, 1, 1: 53–61.

Strauss, A. L. (1978) *Negotiations: varieties, contexts, processes and social order*. Jossey-Bass, London.

Street, A. (1992) *Inside Nursing: A Critical Ethnography*. State University of New York Press, Albany, New York.

Sutton, F. and Smith, C. (1995) Advanced nursing practice: new ideas and new perspectives. *Journal of Advanced Nursing*, 21, 1037–1043.

Svensson, R. (1996) The interplay between doctors and nurses – a negotiated order perspective. *Sociology of Health and Illness*, 18: 379–398.

Swan, B. A. (1993) NPs and anaesthesiologists: a collaborative practice mode. *The Nurse Practitioner: American Journal of Primary Care*, 18: 10–13.

Sweet, S. J. and Norman, I. J. (1995) The doctor-nurse relationship: a selective literature review. *Journal of Advanced Nursing*, 22, 1: 165–170.

Taylor, C. (1997) Problem solving in clinical nursing practice. *Journal of Advanced Nursing*, 26: 329–336.

Taylor, J. S. (1996) Collaborative practice within the intensive care unit: a deconstruction. *Intensive and Critical Care Nursing*, 12: 64–70.

Temkin-Greener, H. (1983) Interpersonal perspectives on teamwork in health care: a case study. *Milbank Memorial Fund Quarterly*, 61, 4: 641–658.

Thomas, K. (1976) Conflict and conflict management. In *Handbook of Industrial and Organisational Psychology*. Dunnette, M., ed. Rand McNally, Chicago.

Thompson, C., McCaughan, D., Cullum, N., Sheldon, T. and Thompson, D. (2000) Nurses' use of research information in clinical decision making. A descriptive and analytical study – final report. *Lancet*, NCC SDO.

Thompson, C. and Dowding, D. (2002) *Clinical Decision Making and Judgement in Nursing*. Harcourt Health Sciences, Oxford.

Thompson, D. R. and Webster, R. A. (1986) The clinical nurse specialist in critical care. *Nurse Practitioner*, 1: 236–241.

Traynor, M. (1996) A literary approach to managerial discourse after the NHS reforms, *Sociology of Health and Illness*, 18, 3: 315–340.

Traynor, M. (1999) *Managerialism and Nursing*. Routledge, London.

Trevillion, S. (1995) *Competent to Collaborate*. CAIPE Bulletin, 10, 6.

Tuckett, D. Boulton, M. Olson, C. and Williams, A. (1985) *Meetings between Experts*. Tavistock, London.

Turner, B. S. (1986) The vocabulary of complaints: nursing, professionalism and job context. *The Australian and New Zealand Journal of Sociology*, 22, 3: 368–386.

United Kingdom Central Council for Nursing, Midwifery and Health Visiting (1986) *A New Preparation for Practice*. UKCC, London.

United Kingdom Central Council for Nursing, Midwifery and Health Visiting (1992a) *The Code of Professional Conduct*. UKCC London.

United Kingdom Central Council for Nursing, Midwifery and Health Visiting (1992b) *The Scope of Professional Practice*. UKCC London.

United Kingdom Central Council for Nursing, Midwifery and Health Visiting (1994) *The Future of Professional Practice: The Council's Standards for Education and Practice Following Registration*. UKCC London.

United Kingdom Central Council for Nursing, Midwifery and Health Visiting (1997) *UKCC Position on Advanced Practice*. (Press statement 8/1997). UKCC London.

van Maanen, J., Dabbs, J. M. and Faulkner, R. R. (1982) *Varieties of Qualitative Research*. Sage, Beverly Hills.

van Maanen, M. (1990) *Researching the Lived Experience: Human Science for Active Sensitive Pedagogy*. Althouse Press, Ontario.

Viney, C. (1996) A phenomenological study of ethical decision making experiences among senior intensive care nurses and doctors concerning withdrawal of treatment. *Nursing in Critical Care*, 1, 4: 182–187.

Walby, S. and Greenwall, J. (1994) *Medicine and Nursing in a Changing Health Service*. Sage, London.

Wallace, M. and Gough, P. (1995) The UKCC's criteria for specialist and advanced practice. *British Journal of Nursing*, 4, 16: 939–941.

Walsh, M. and Ford, P. (1989) We always do it this way. *Nursing Times*, 85, 41: 26–35.

Walt, G. (1994) *Health Policy: An Introduction to Power and Process*. Zed Books, London.

Walt, G. and Gilson, L. (1994) Reforming the health sector in developing countries: the central role of policy analysis. *Health Policy and Planning*, 9, 4: 353–370.

Watson, J. (1979) *Nursing: The Philosophy and Science of Caring*. Little, Brown, Boston.

Webb, A. R. (1996) Medical staffing and training: the United Kingdom perspective. In *Critical Care Standards Audit and Ethics*. Tinker, J., Browne, D. and Sibbald, W. J., eds. Arnold Press, New York.

Webster (1990) *Webster's 9th New Collegiate Dictionary*. Merriam Webster Inc., Springfield, MA.

Weil, M. H., Shubin, H. and Biddle, M. (1964) Shock caused by gram negative micro-organisms, analysis of 169 cases. *Annals of Internal Medicine*, 60: 384–400.

Weiss, S. J. (1983) Role differentiation between nurses and physicians: implications for nursing. *Nursing Research*, 32, 2: 133–139.

Weiss, S. J. and Davis, H. (1985) Validity and reliability of the collaborative practice scales. *Nursing Research*, 34: 299–305.

White, R. (1988) *Political Issues in Nursing: Past, Present and Future*. Vol. 3. John Wiley and Sons, London.

Whyte, W. F. (1981) *Street Corner Society: The Social Structure of an Italian Slum*, 3rd edn. University of Chicago Press, Chicago.

Wicks, D. (1995) Nurses and doctors and discourses of healing. *Australian and New Zealand Journal of Sociology*, 31, 2: 122–139.

Wicks, D. (1998) *Nurses and Doctors at Work: Rethinking Professional Boundaries*. Open University Press, Buckingham.

Williams, A. (1990a) Reading feminism in fieldnotes In *Feminist Praxis Research, Theory and Epistemology in Feminist Sociology*. Stanley, L., ed. Routledge, London.

Williams, A. (1990b) Reflections on the making of an ethnographic text. Studies in Sexual Politics 29, Manchester University Press, Manchester.

Witz, A. (1992) *Profession and Patriarchy*. Routledge, London.

Wolcott, H. (1990) Writing up qualitative research. Qualitative Research Methods Series 20. Sage, Newbury Park, CA.

Wolcott, H. F. (1994) *Transforming Qualitative Data: Description, Analysis, and Interpretation*. Sage, Thousand Oaks, CA.

Wonsetter, L. A. O. (1987) Perceptions of nurse–physicians collaboration in an emergency room setting. PhD thesis. Medical College of Ohio.

Woodrow, P. (1997) Nursing perspectives for intensive care. *Intensive and Critical Care Nursing*, 13: 151–155.

World Health Organisation (2001) World nursing shortage hits critical care. Reported in www.ukcc.org.uk news site.

Zussman, R. (1992) *Intensive Care: Medical Ethics and the Medical Profession*. University of Chicago Press, Chicago.

Index

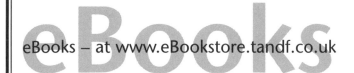